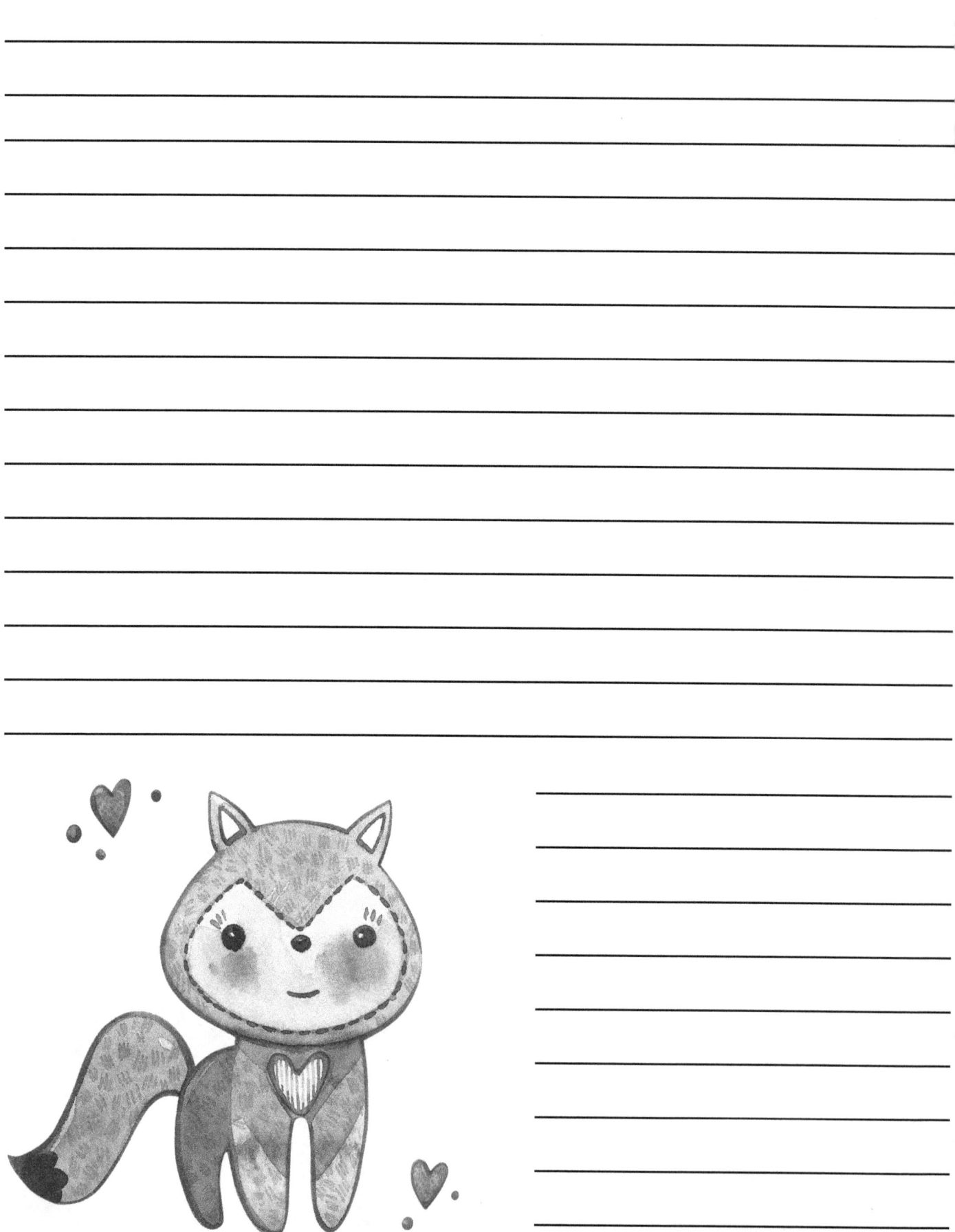

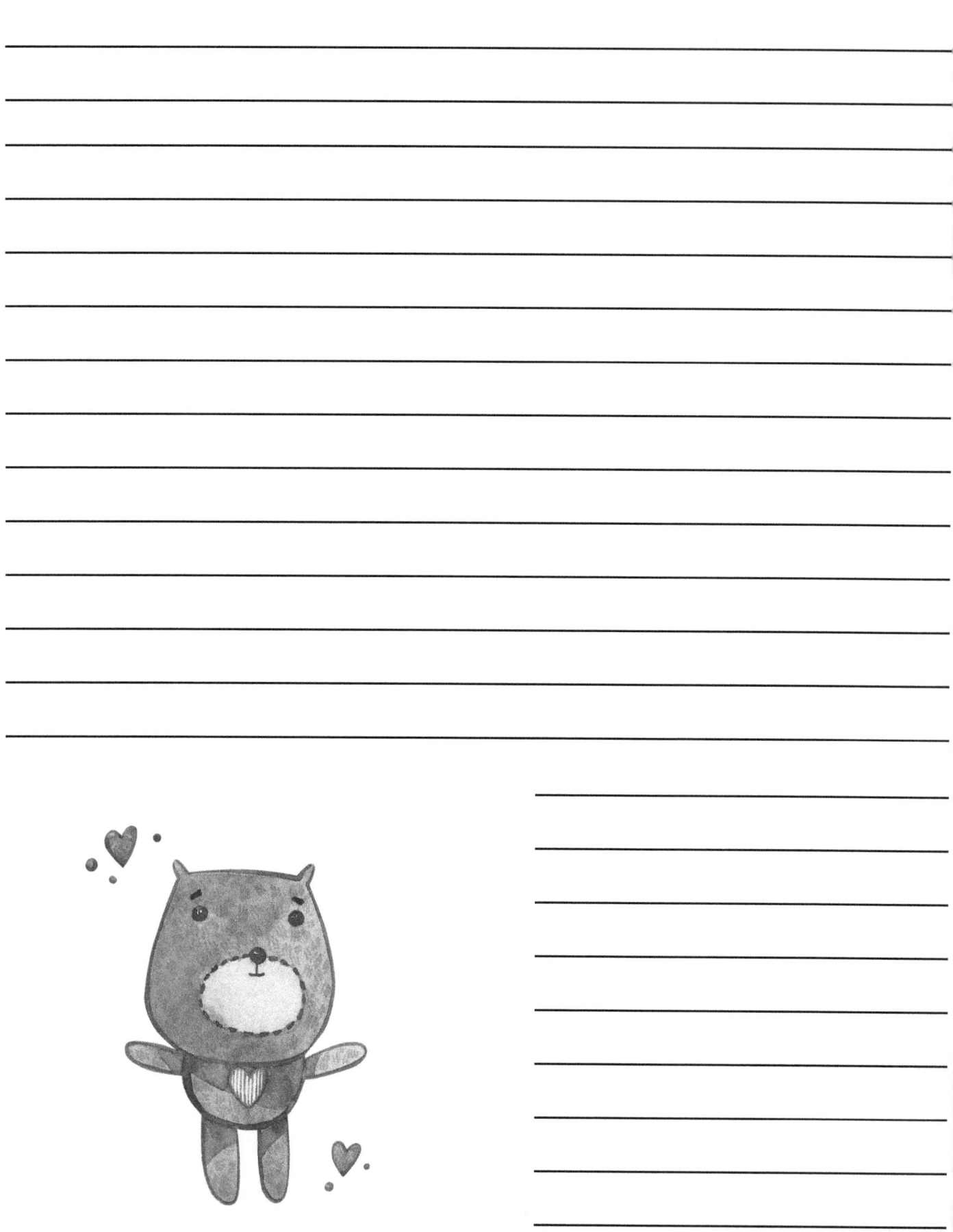

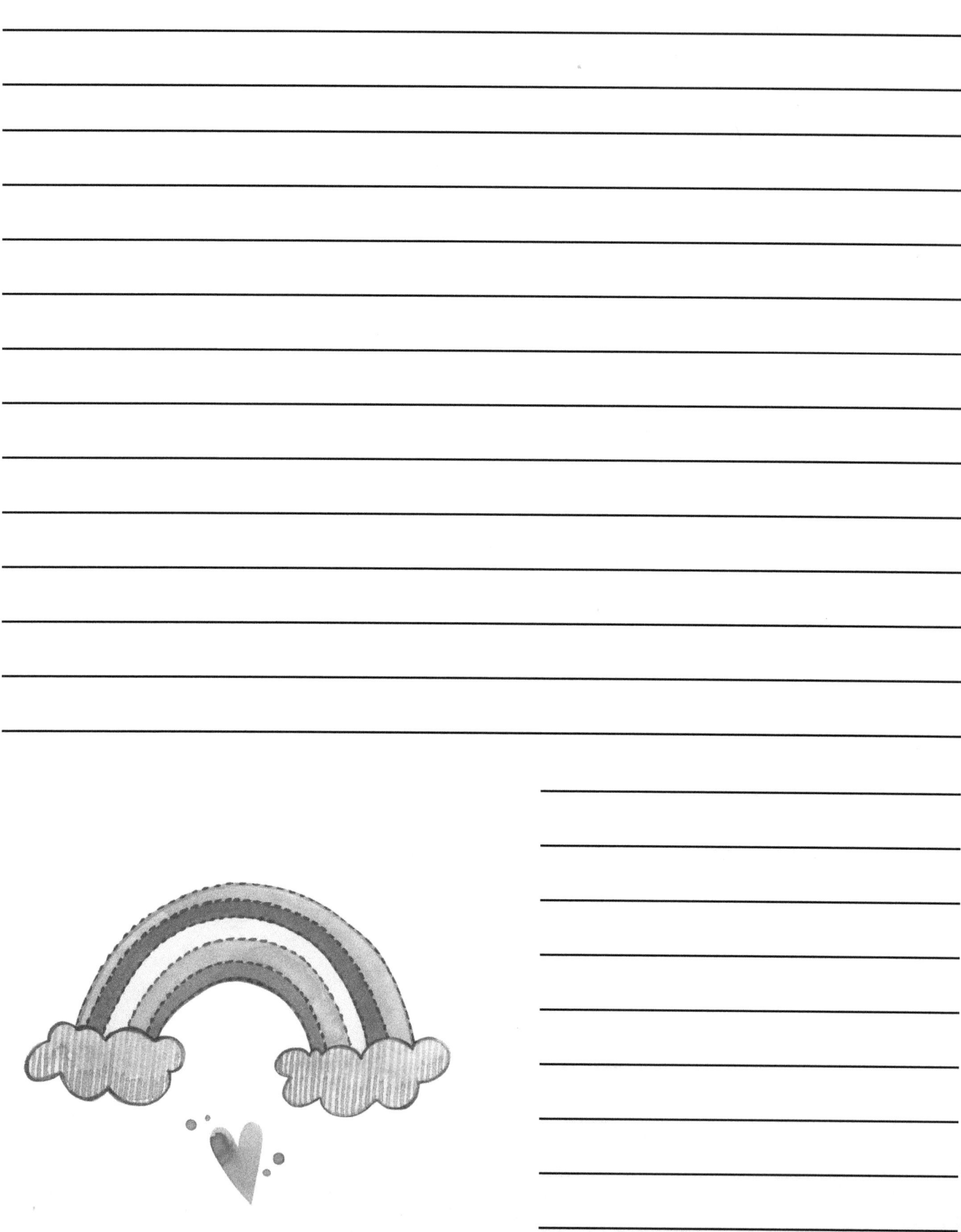

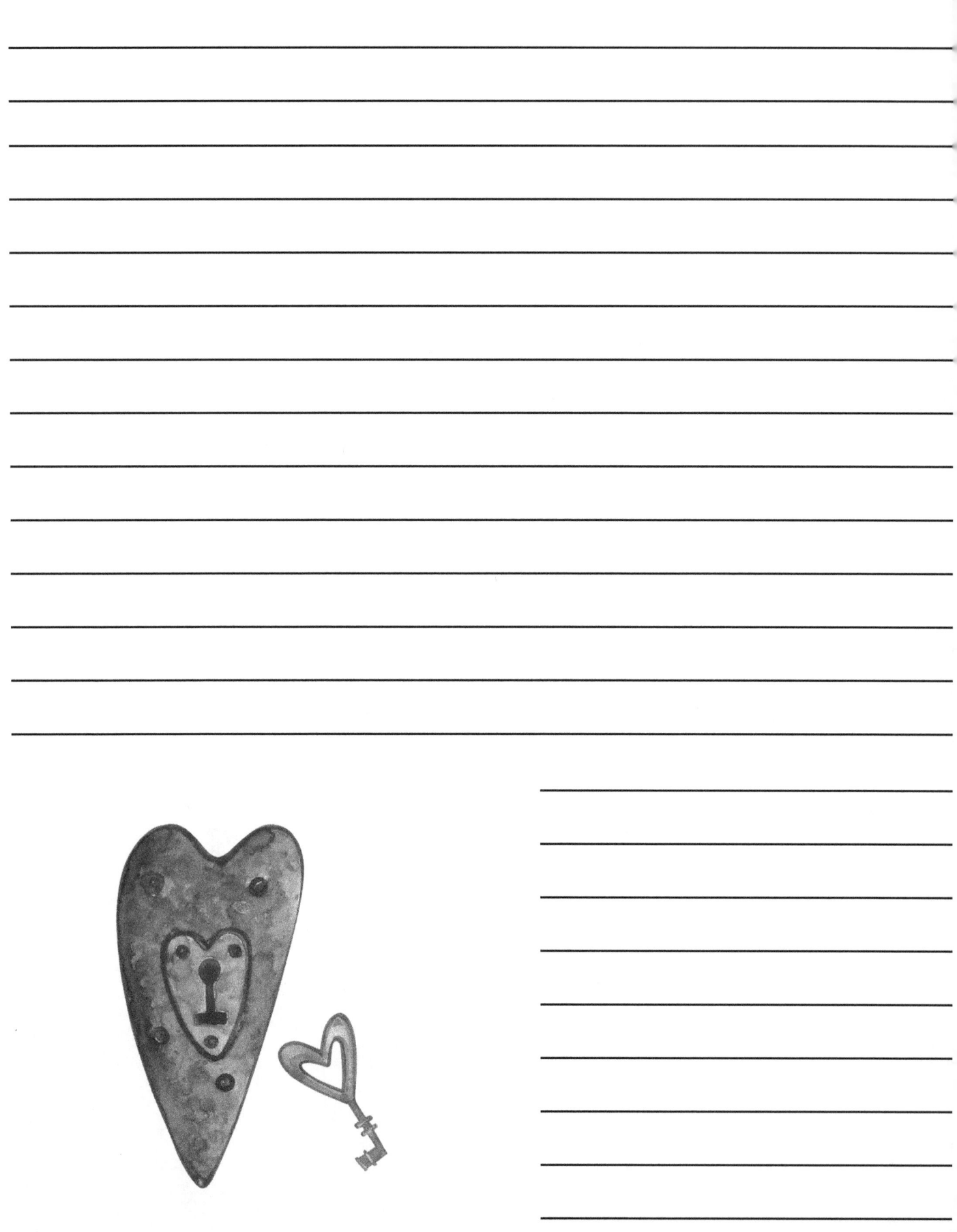

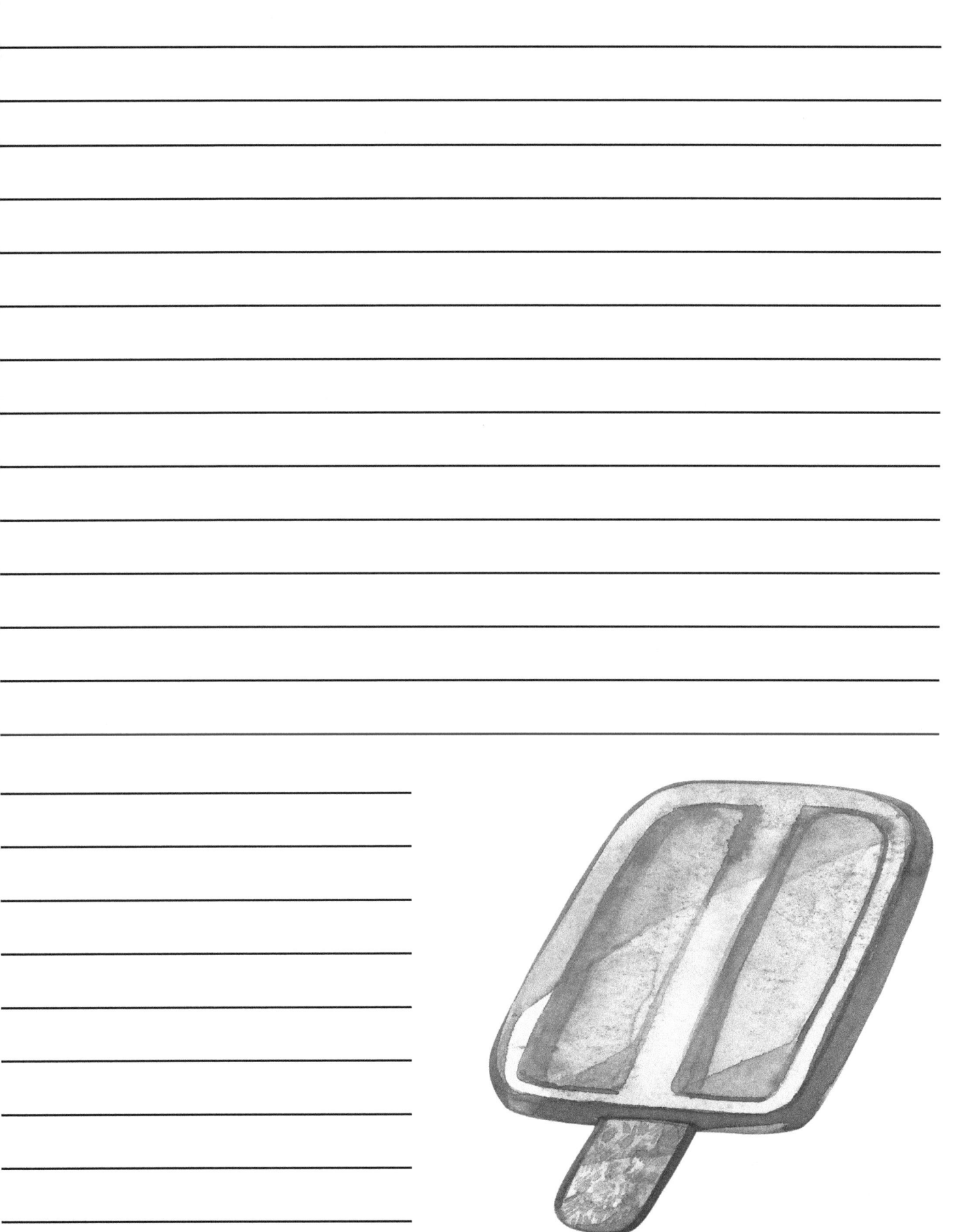

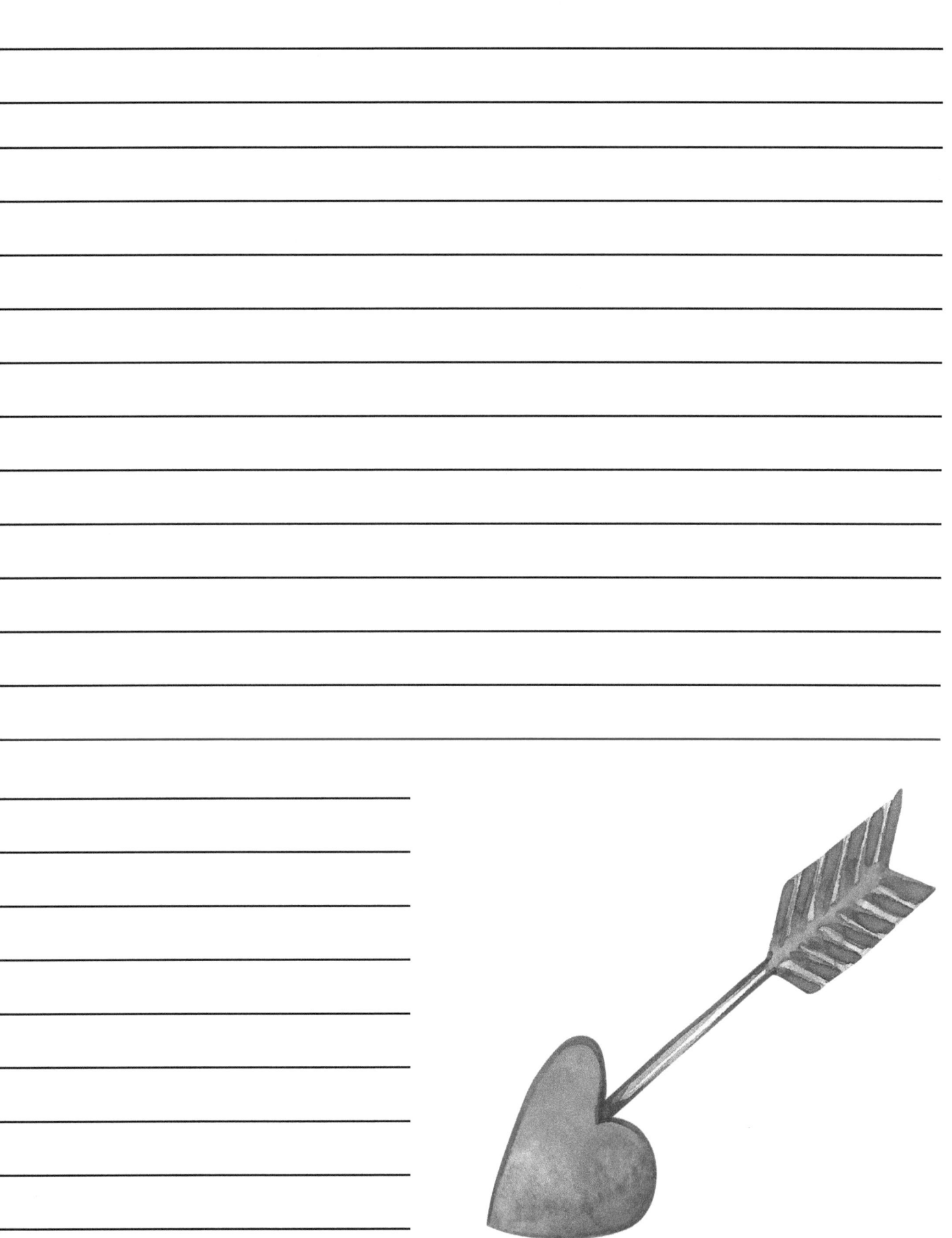

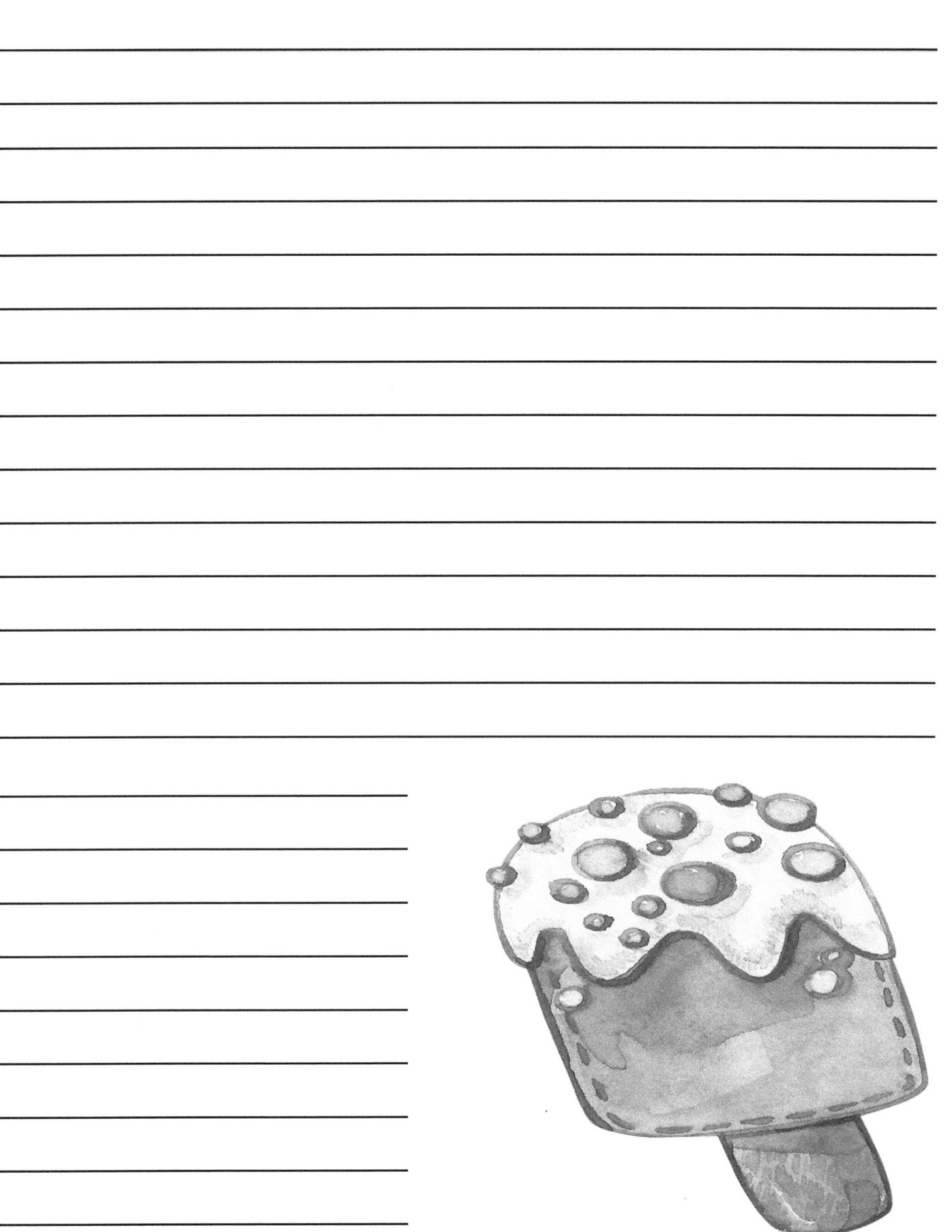

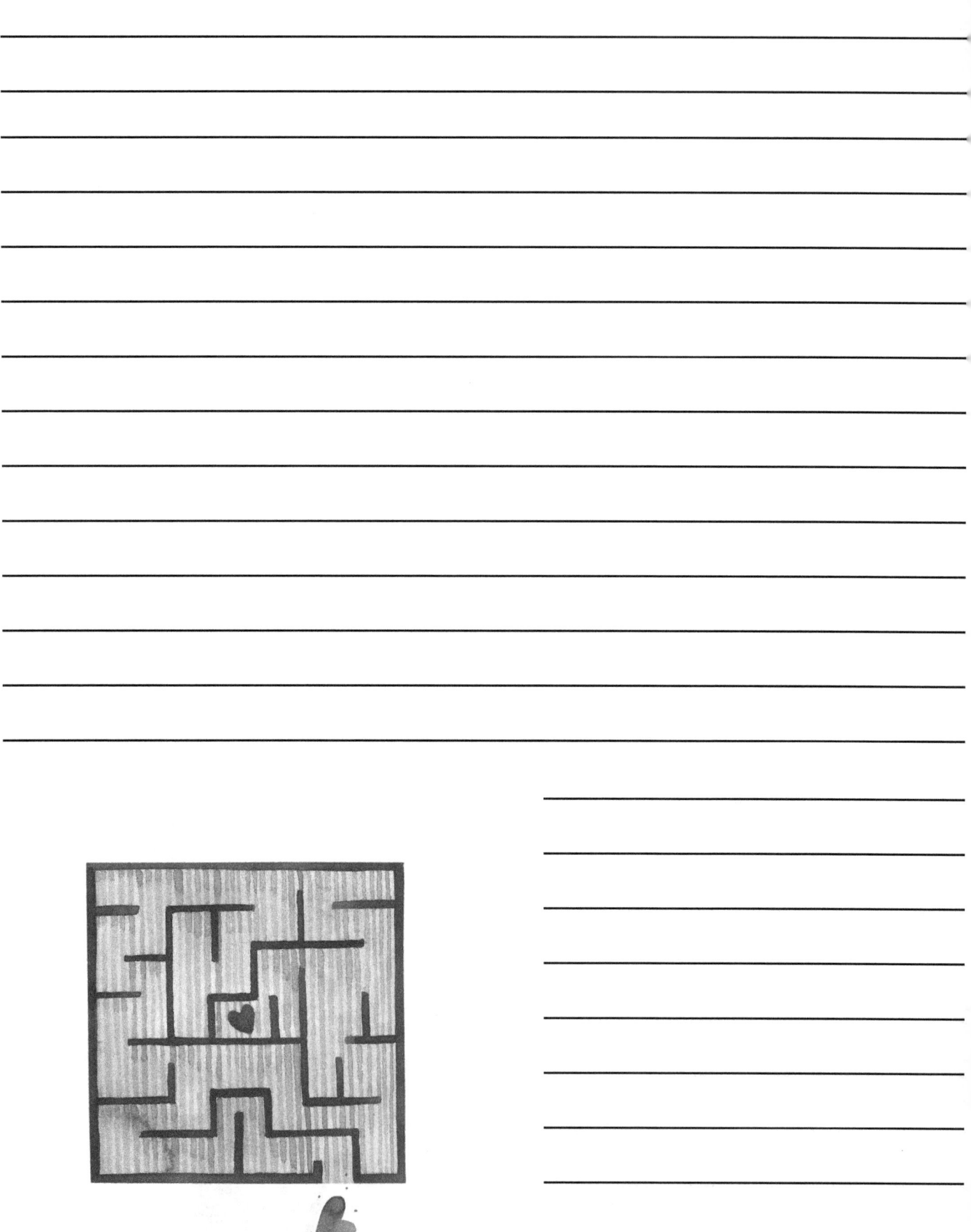

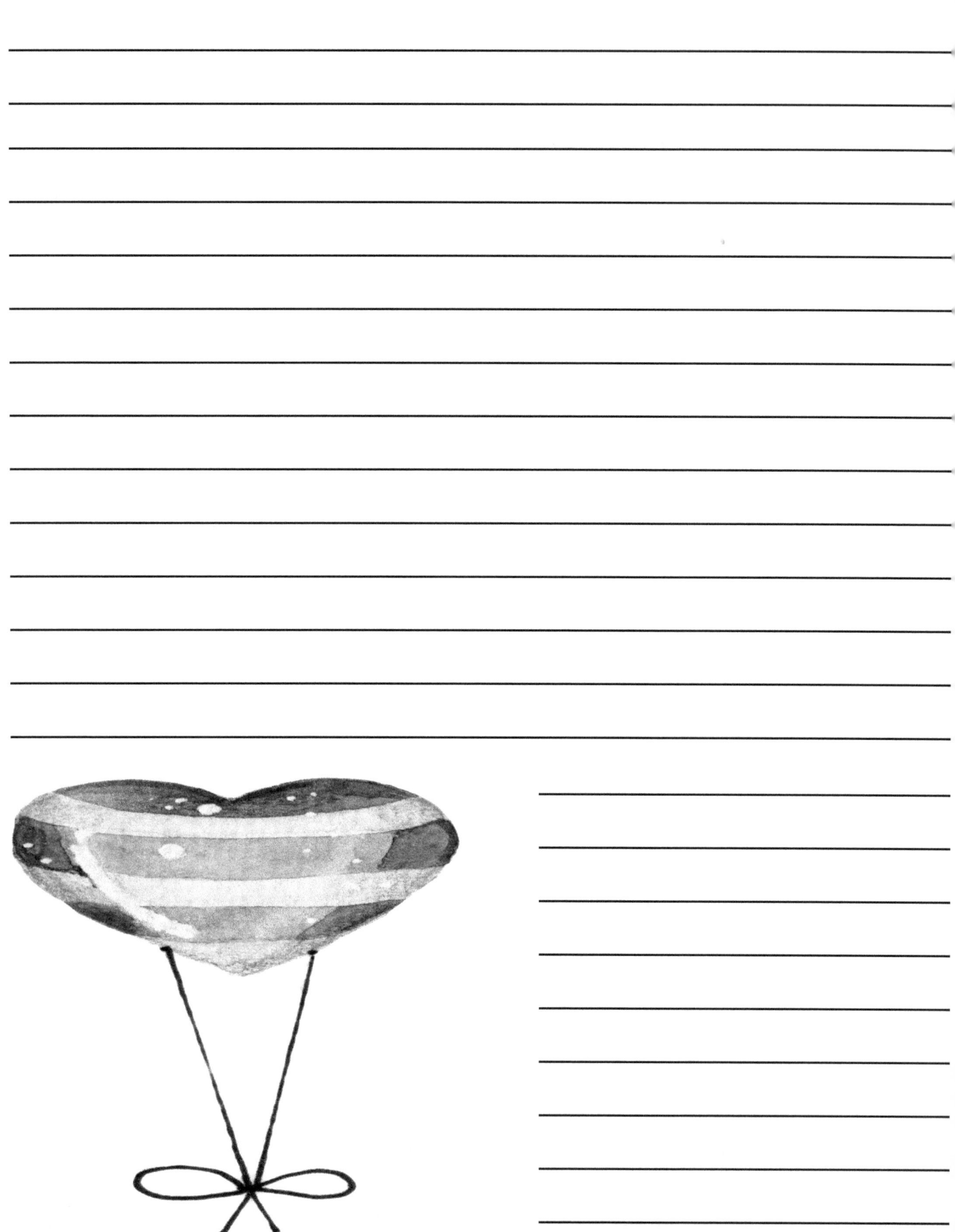

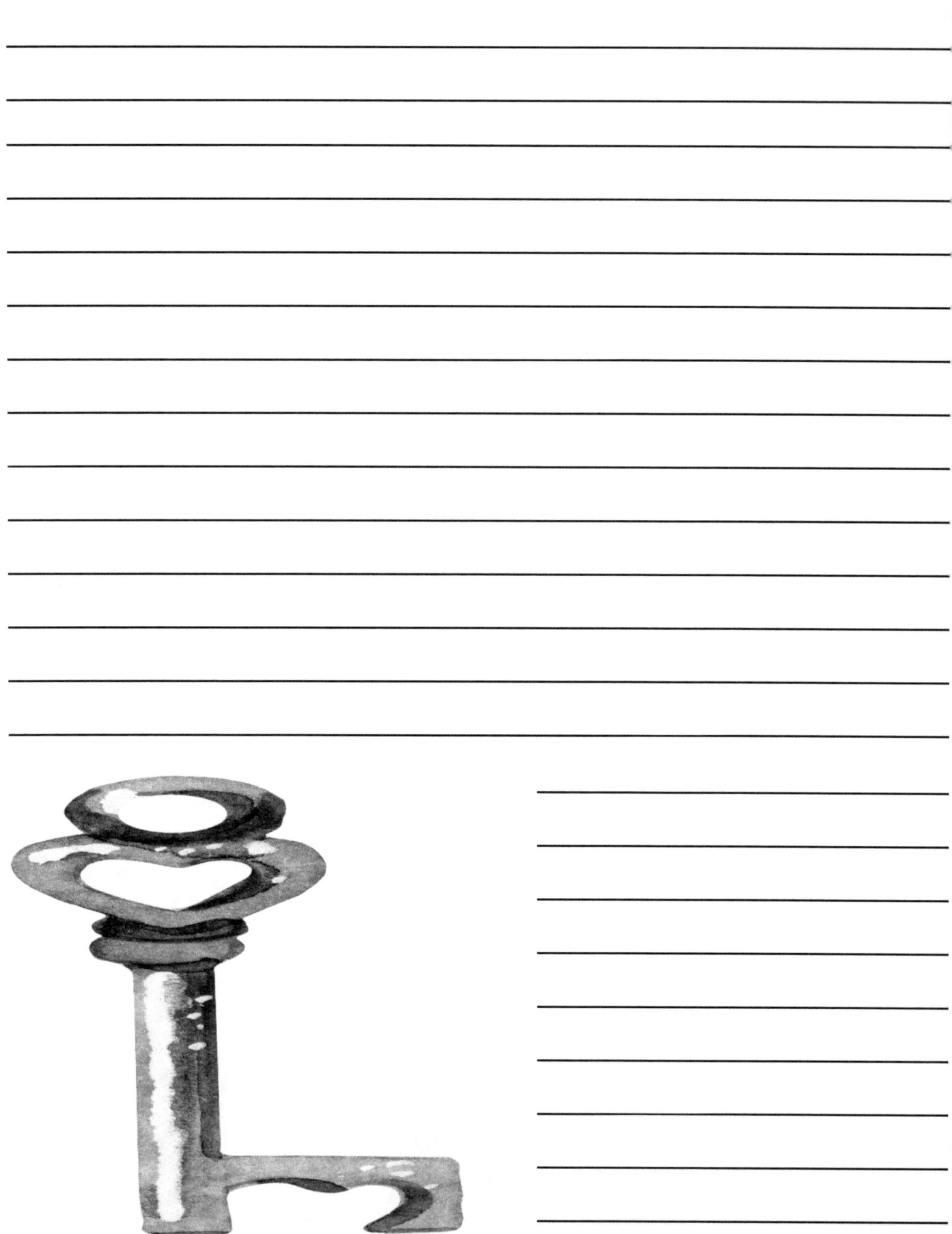

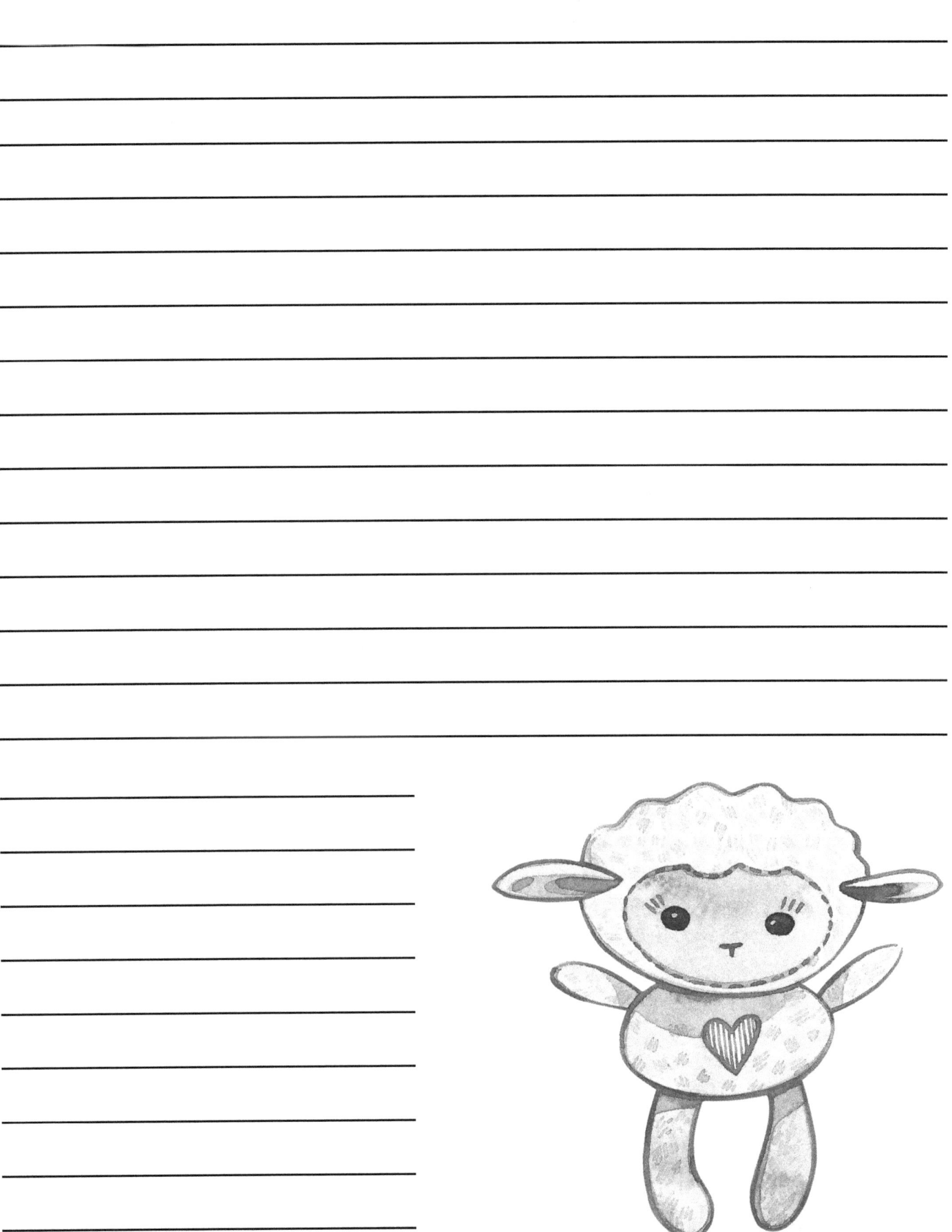

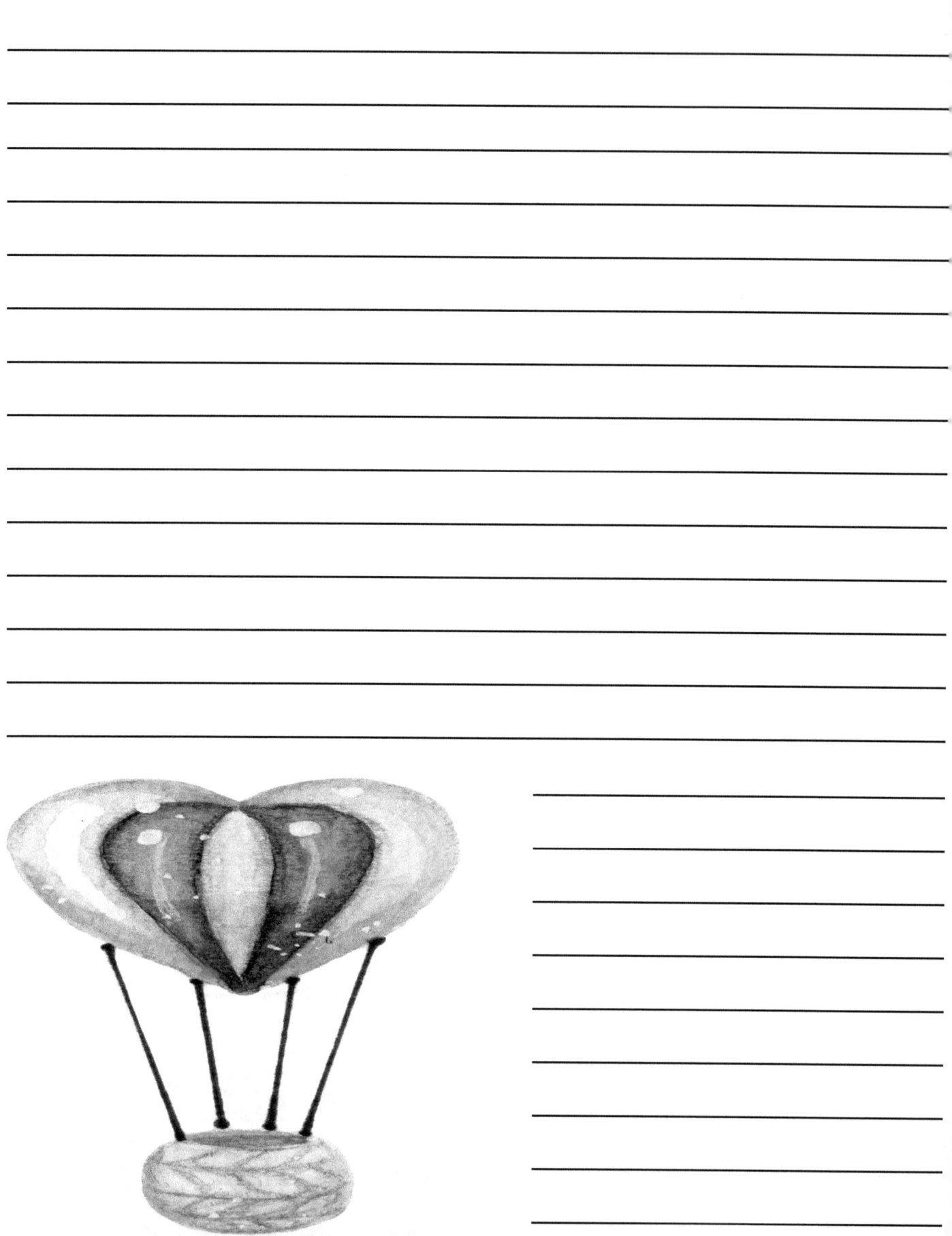

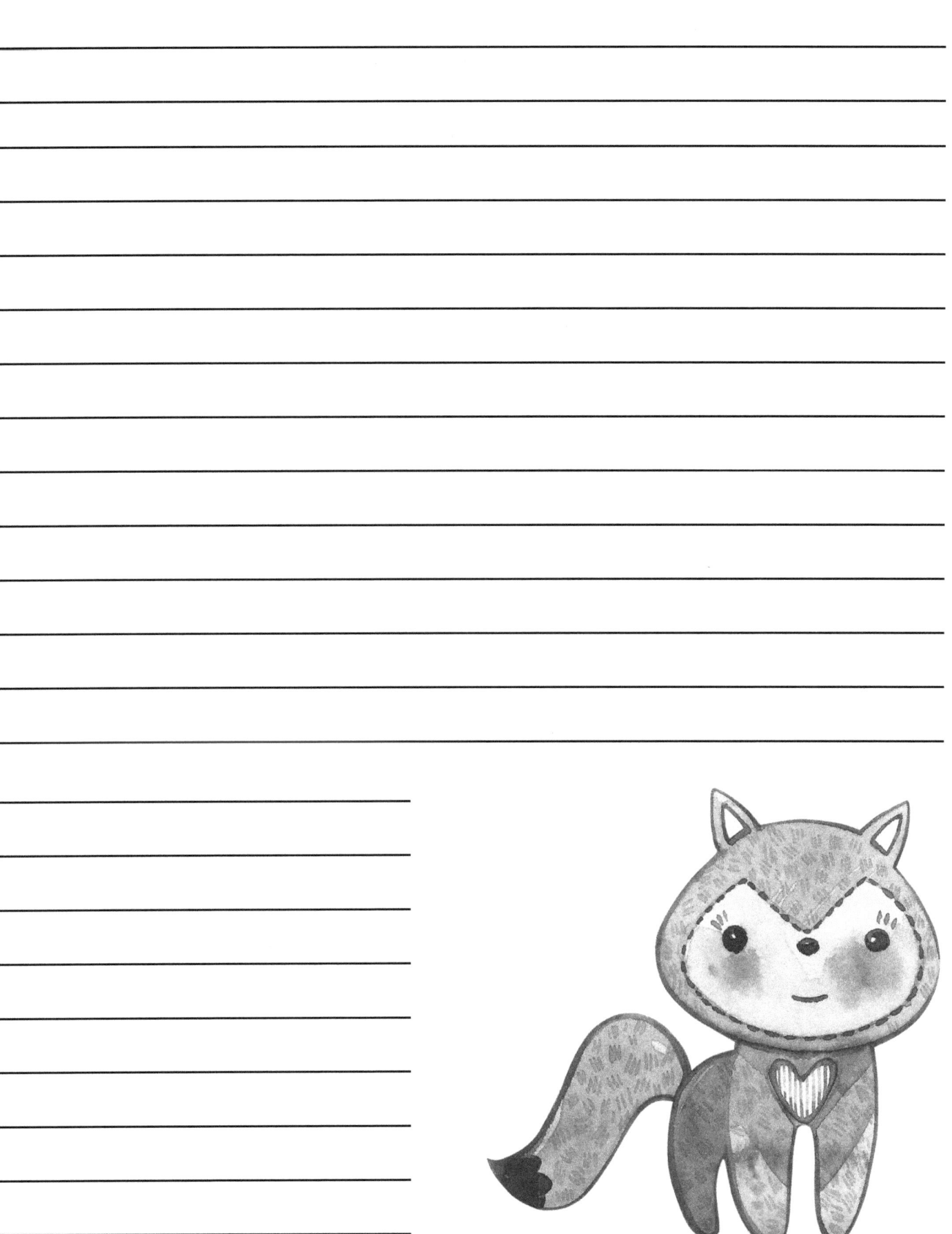

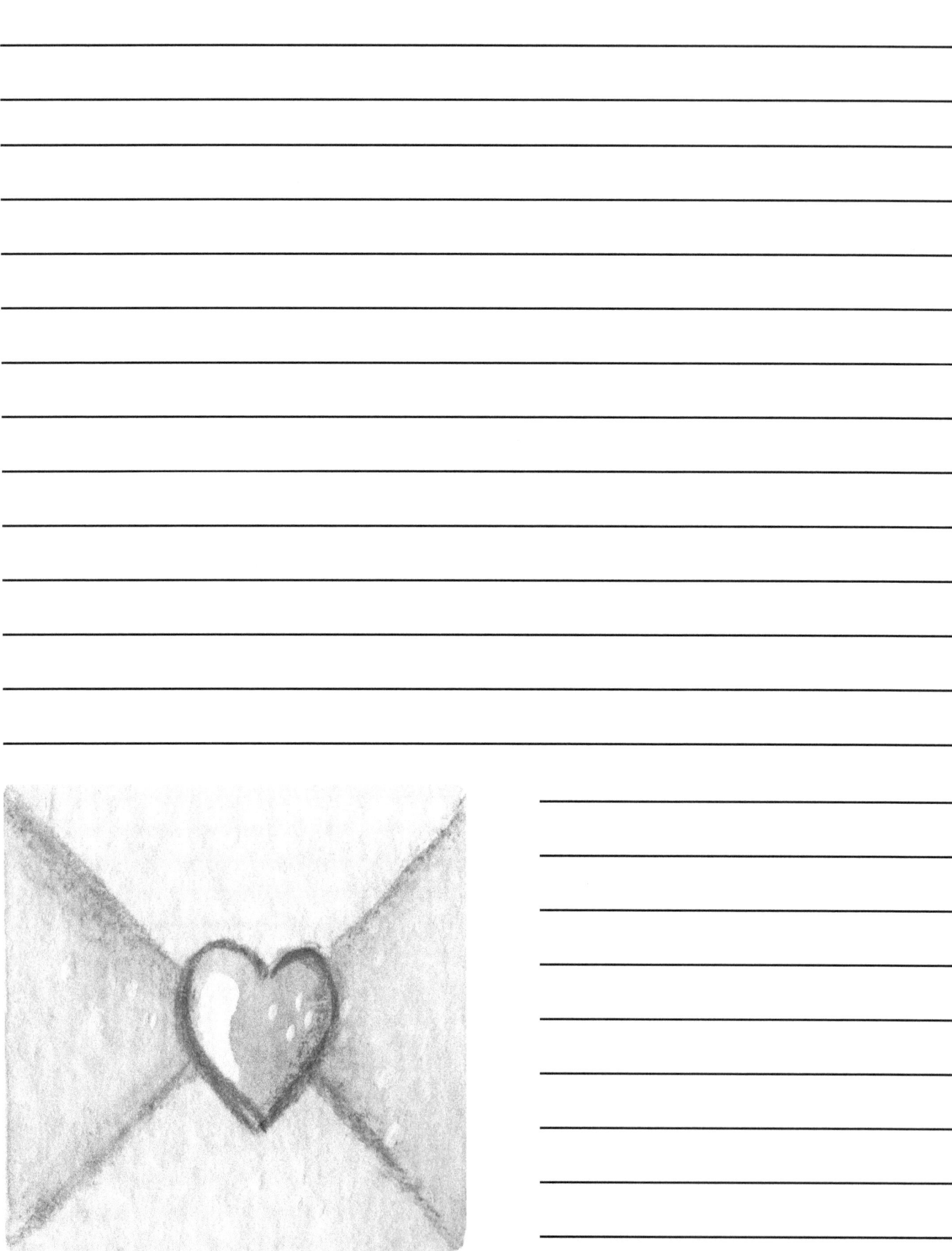

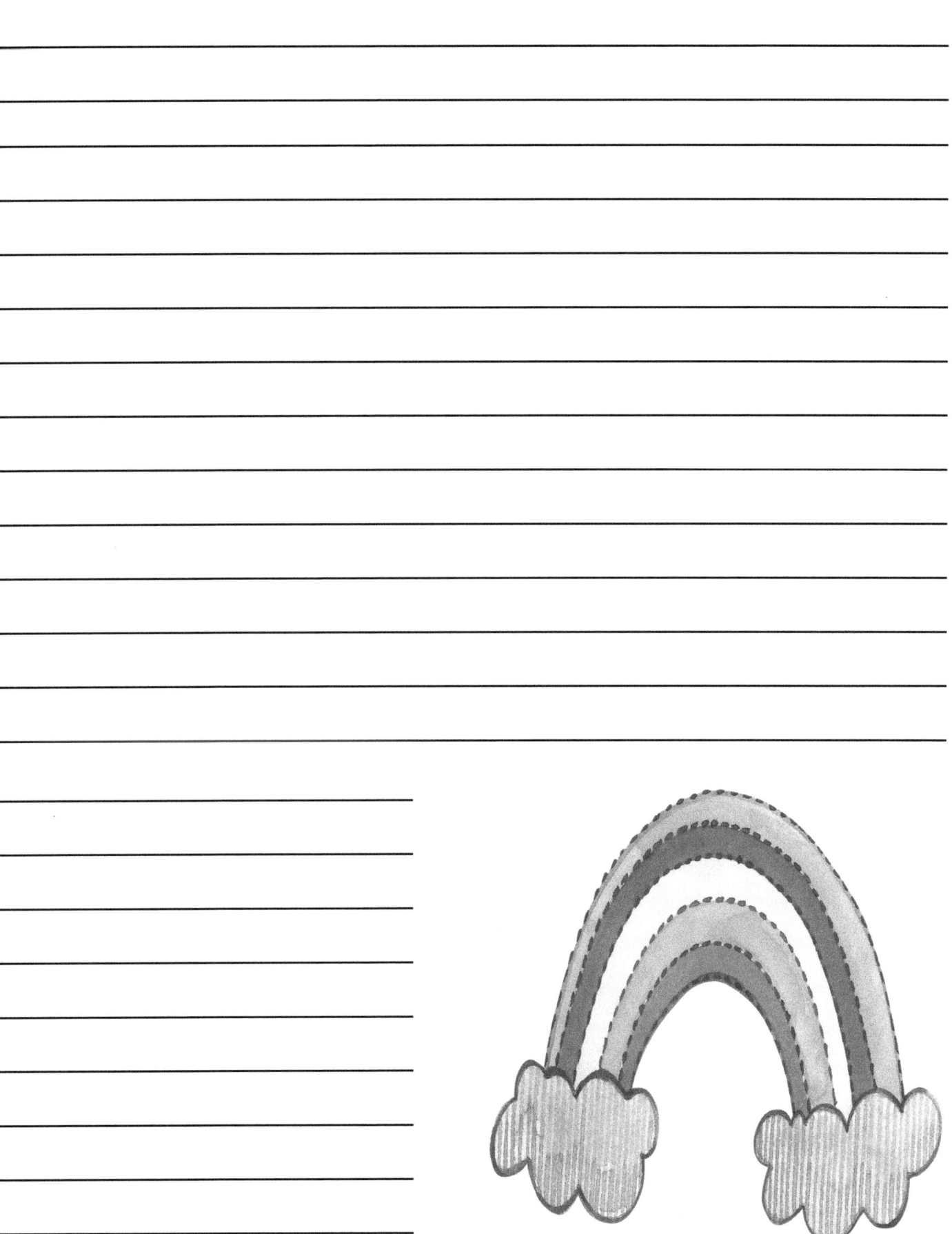

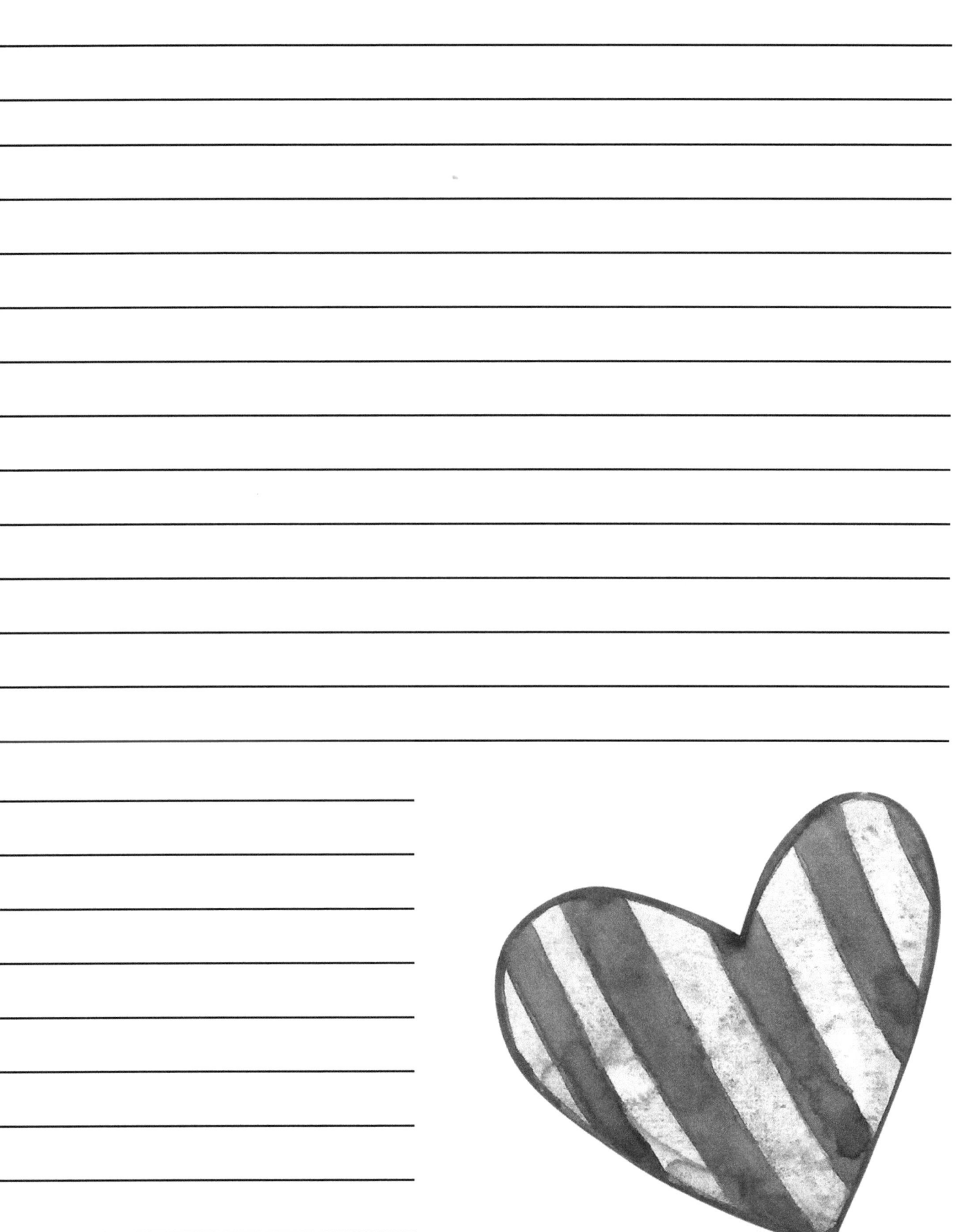

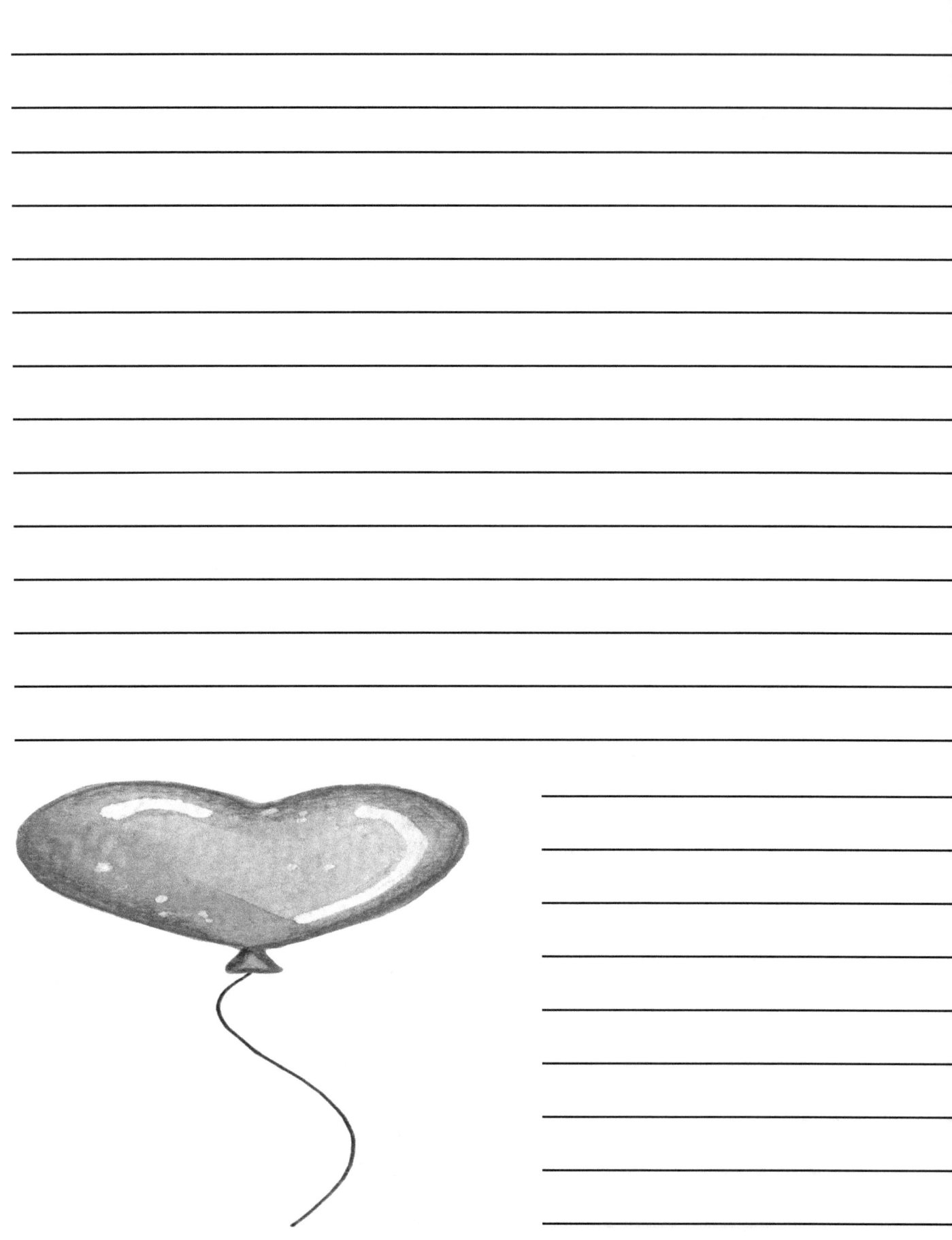

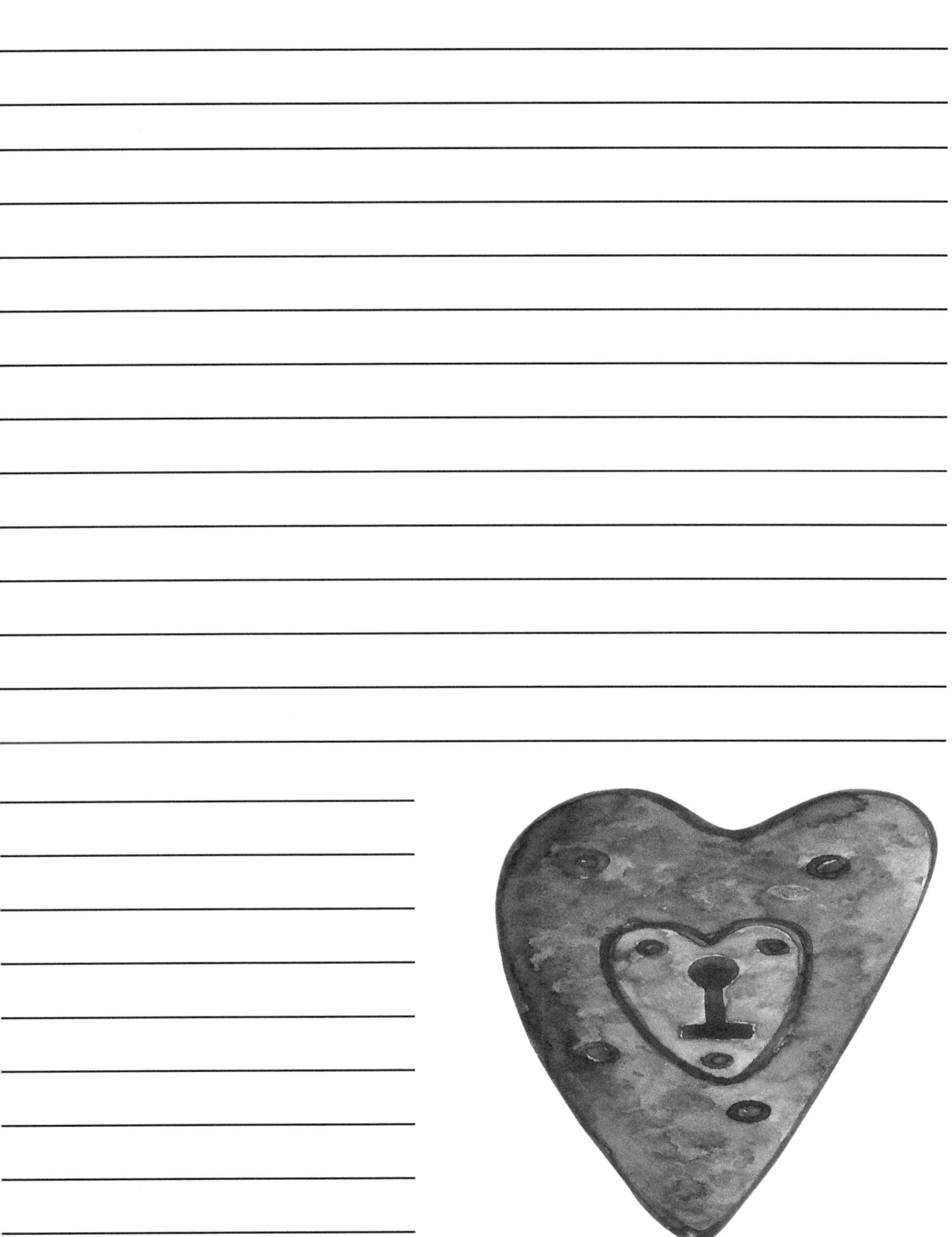

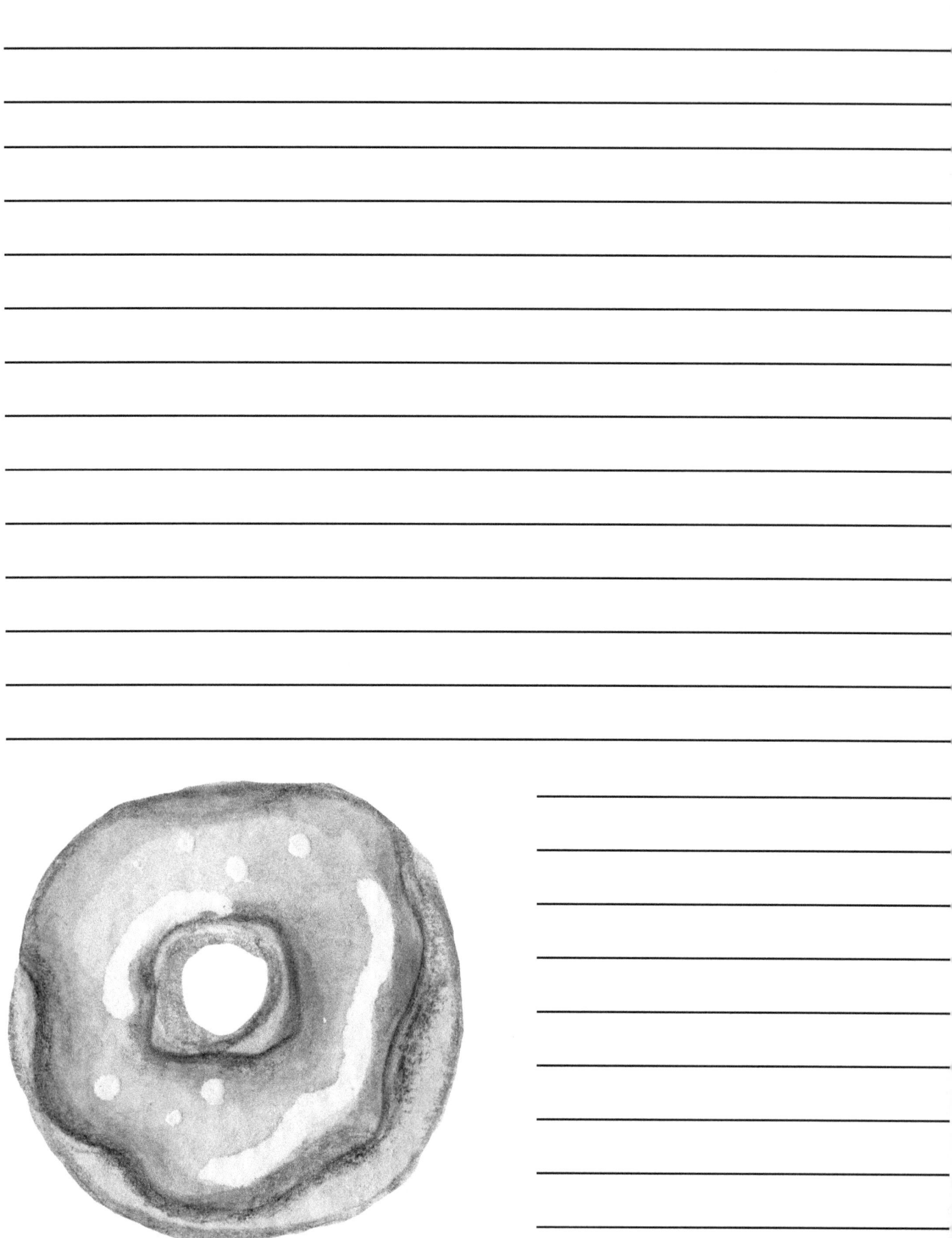

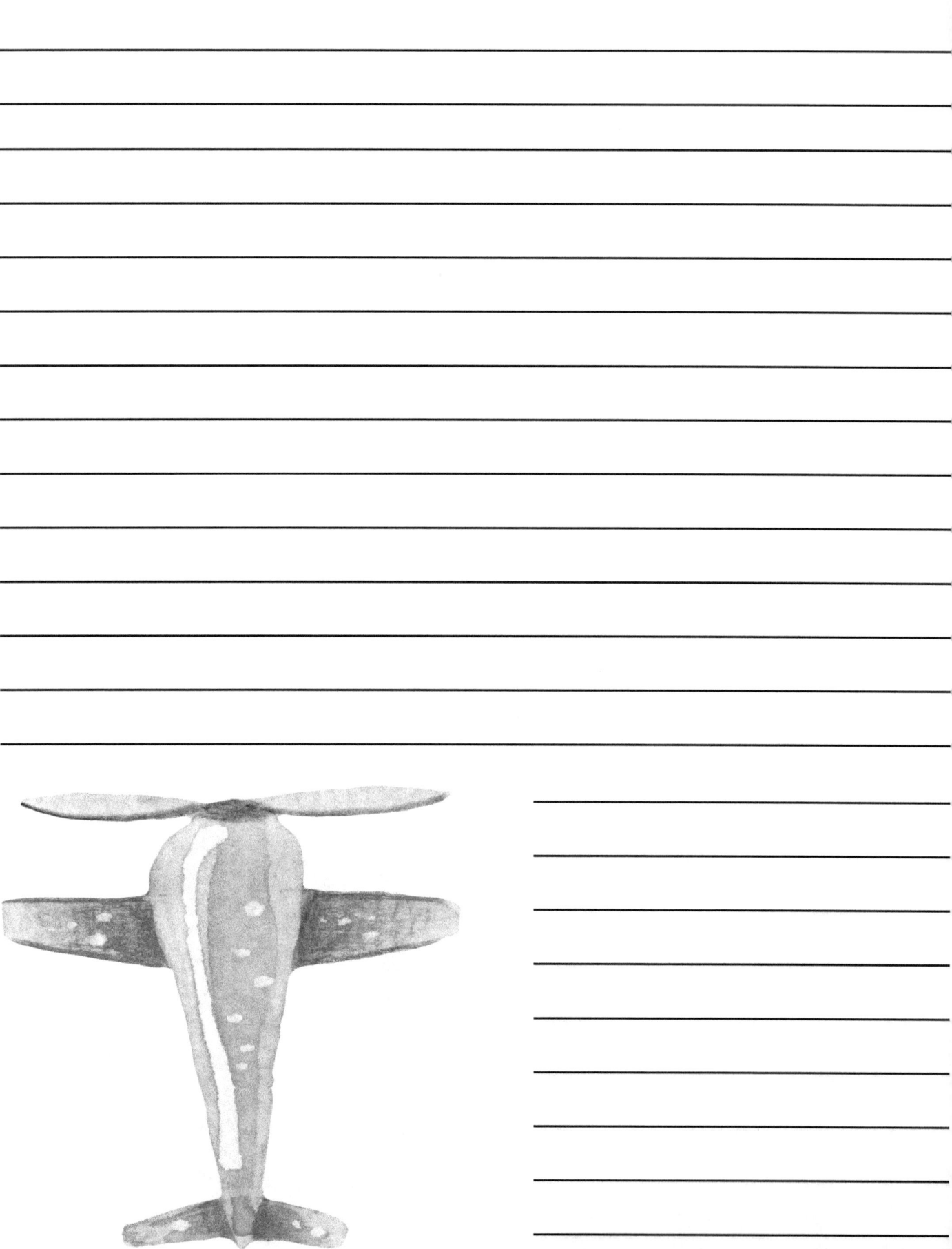

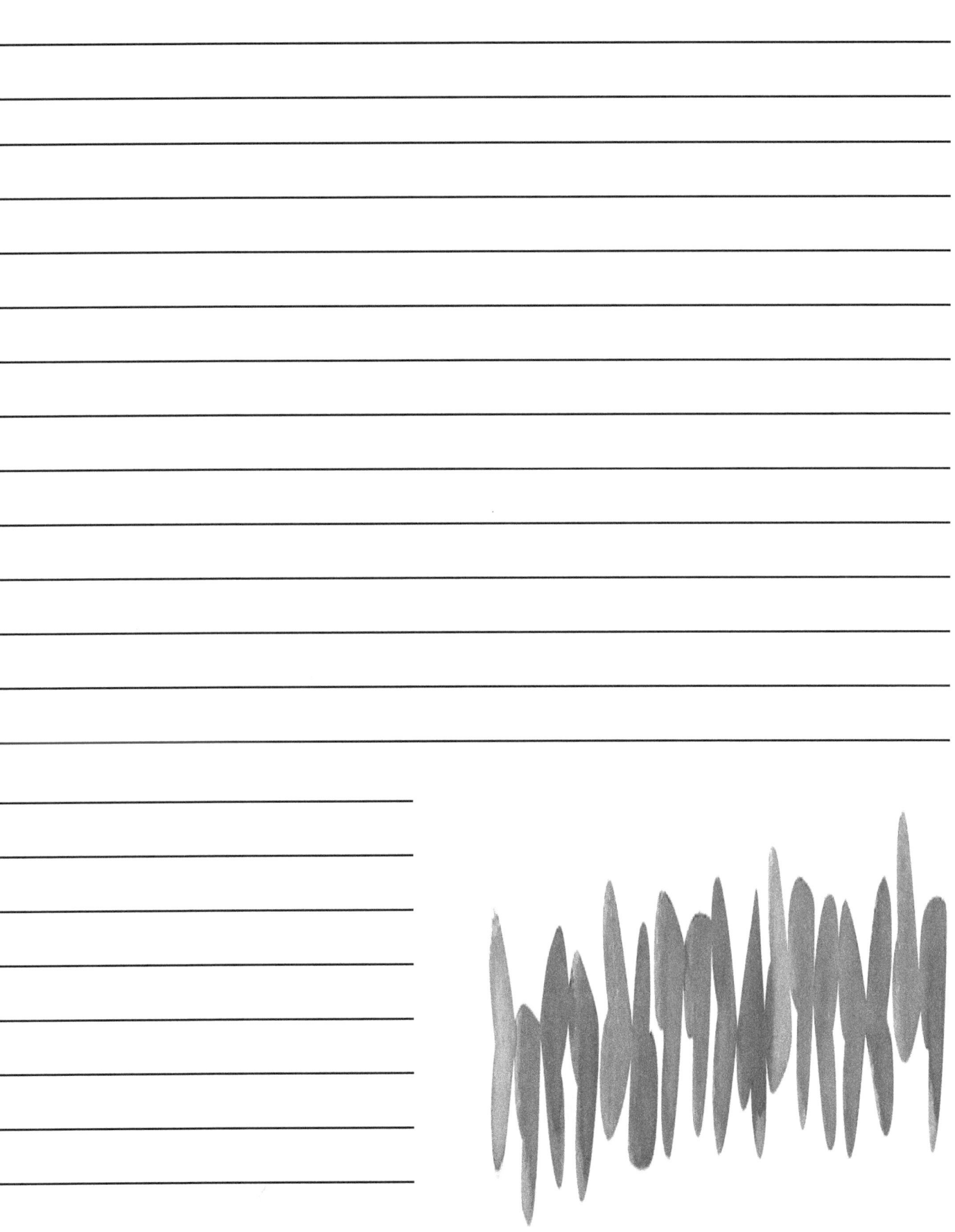

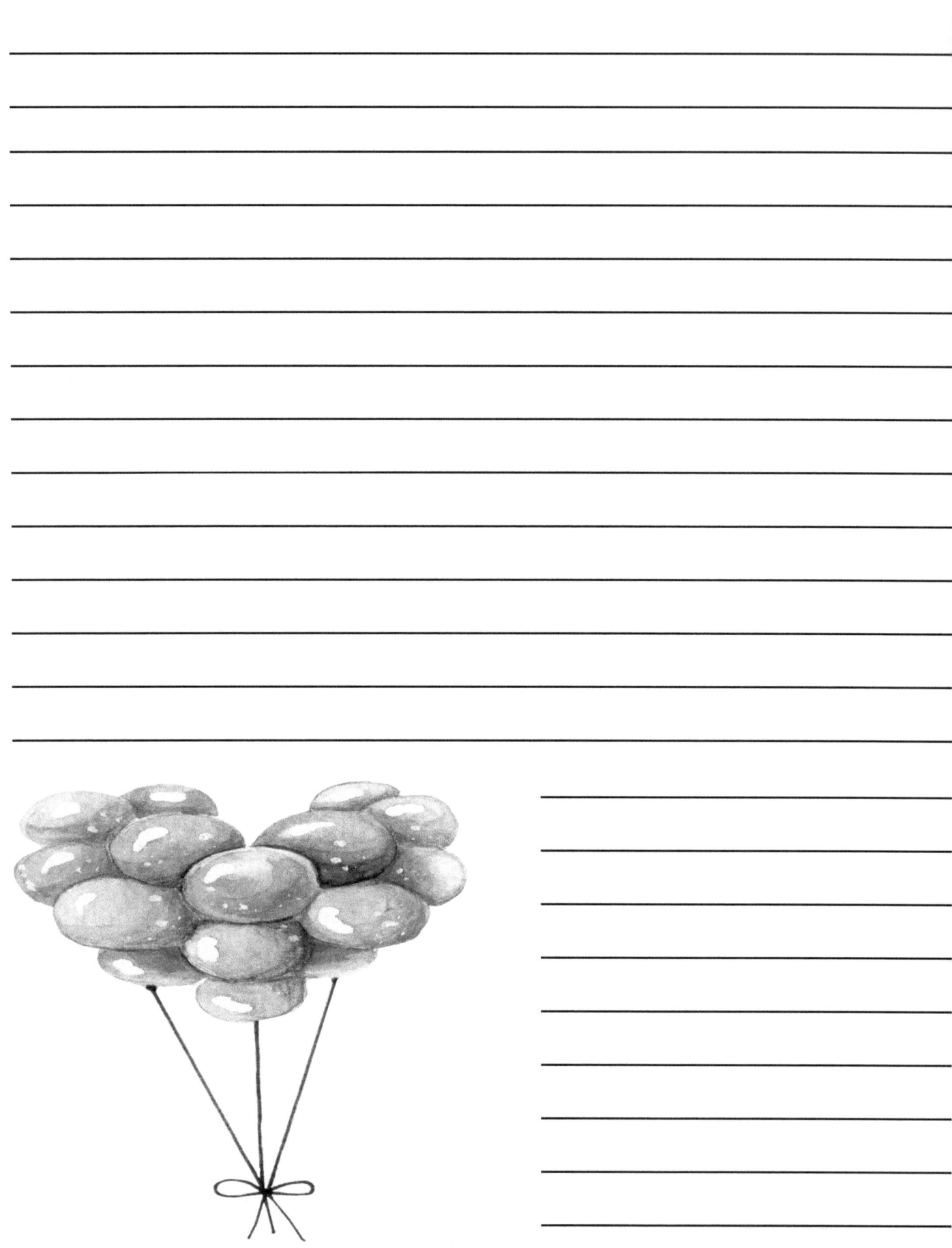

believe IN Love

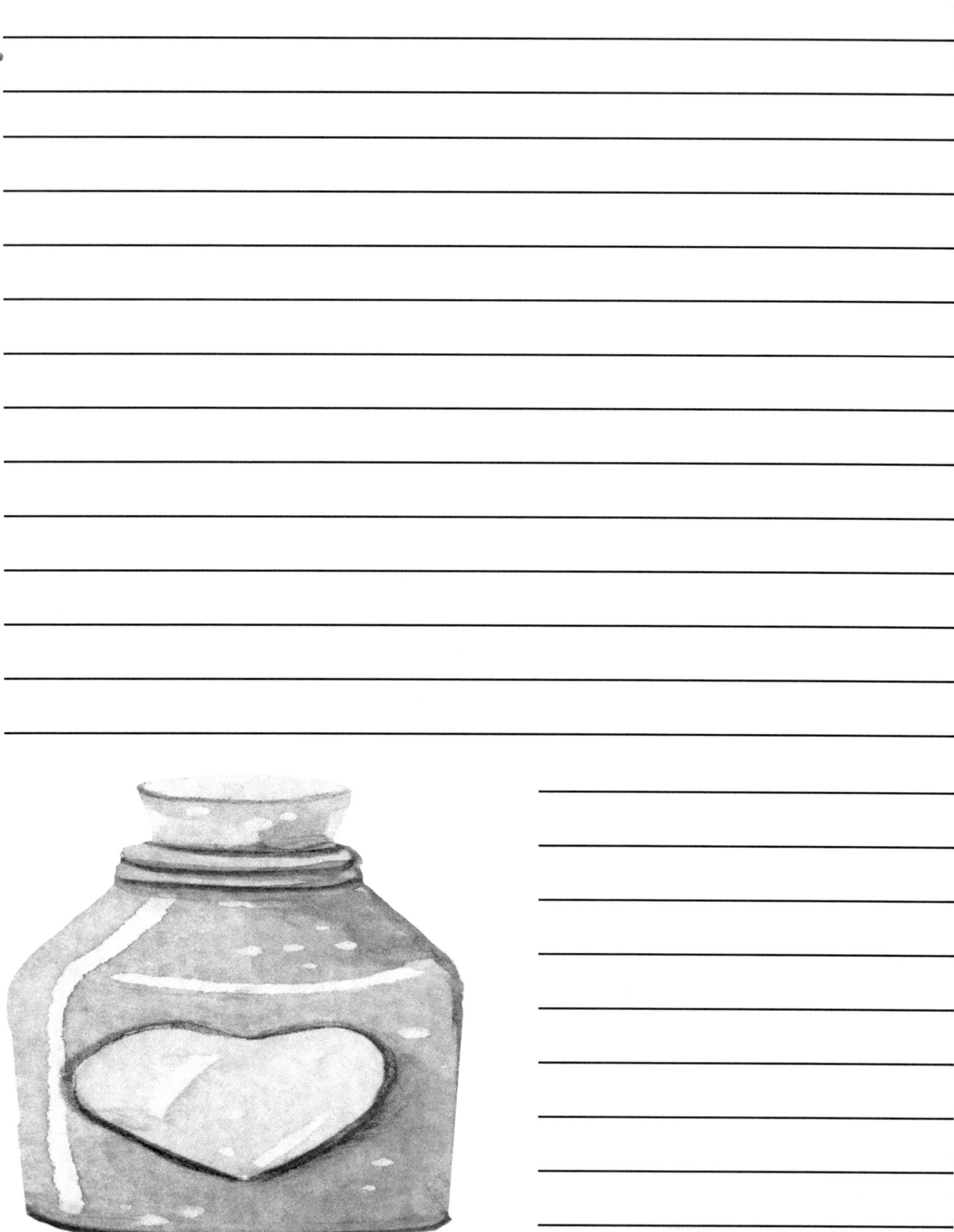

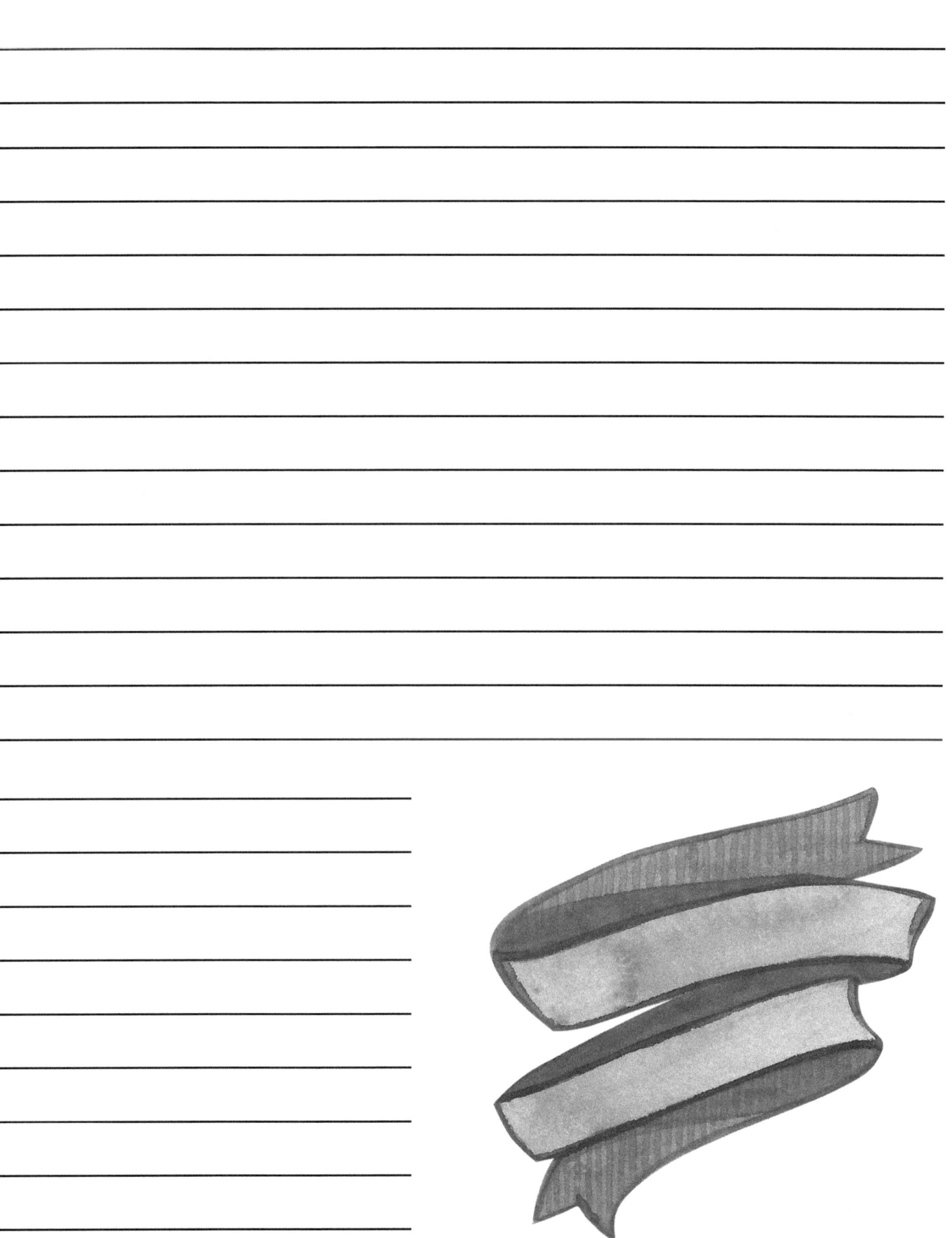

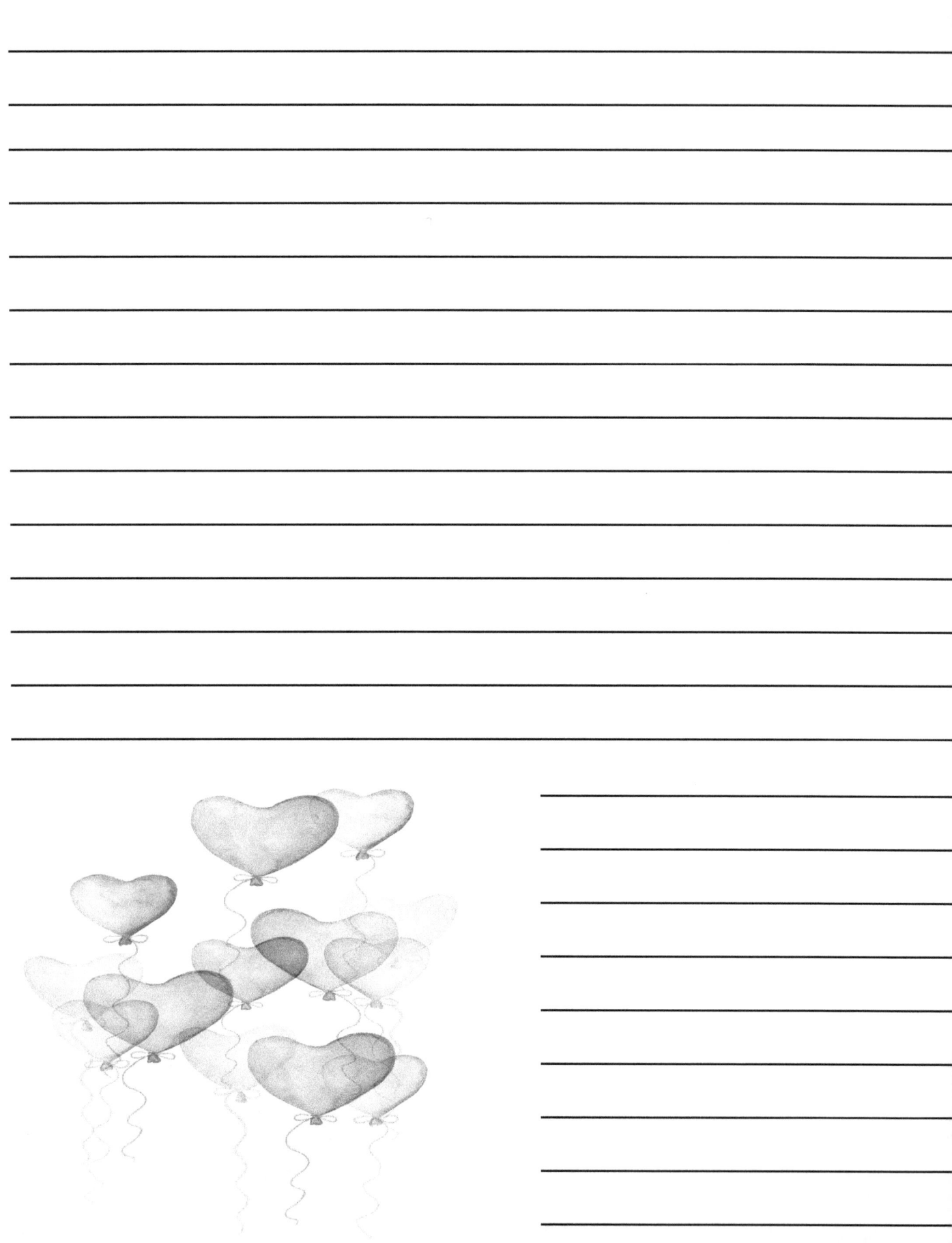

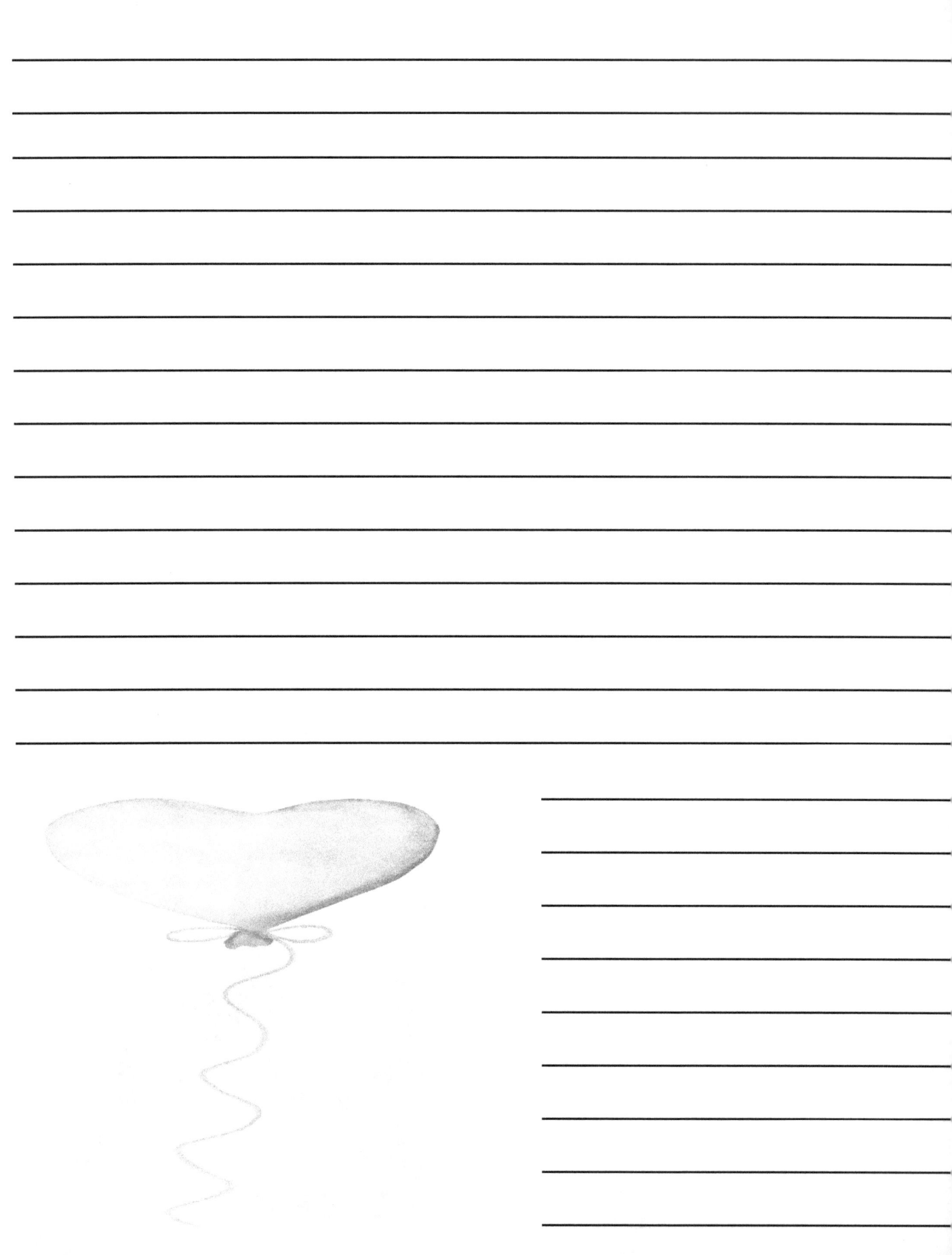

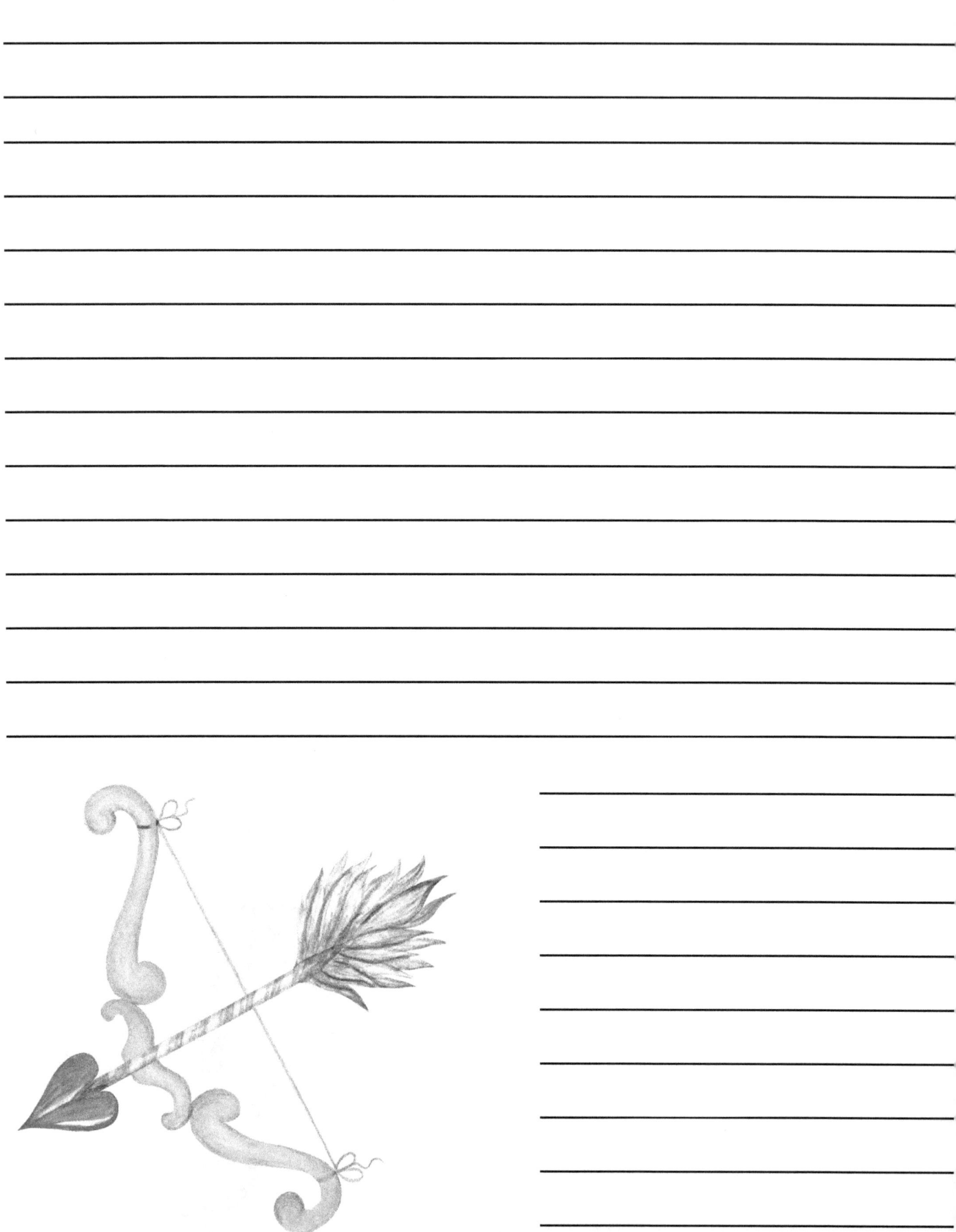

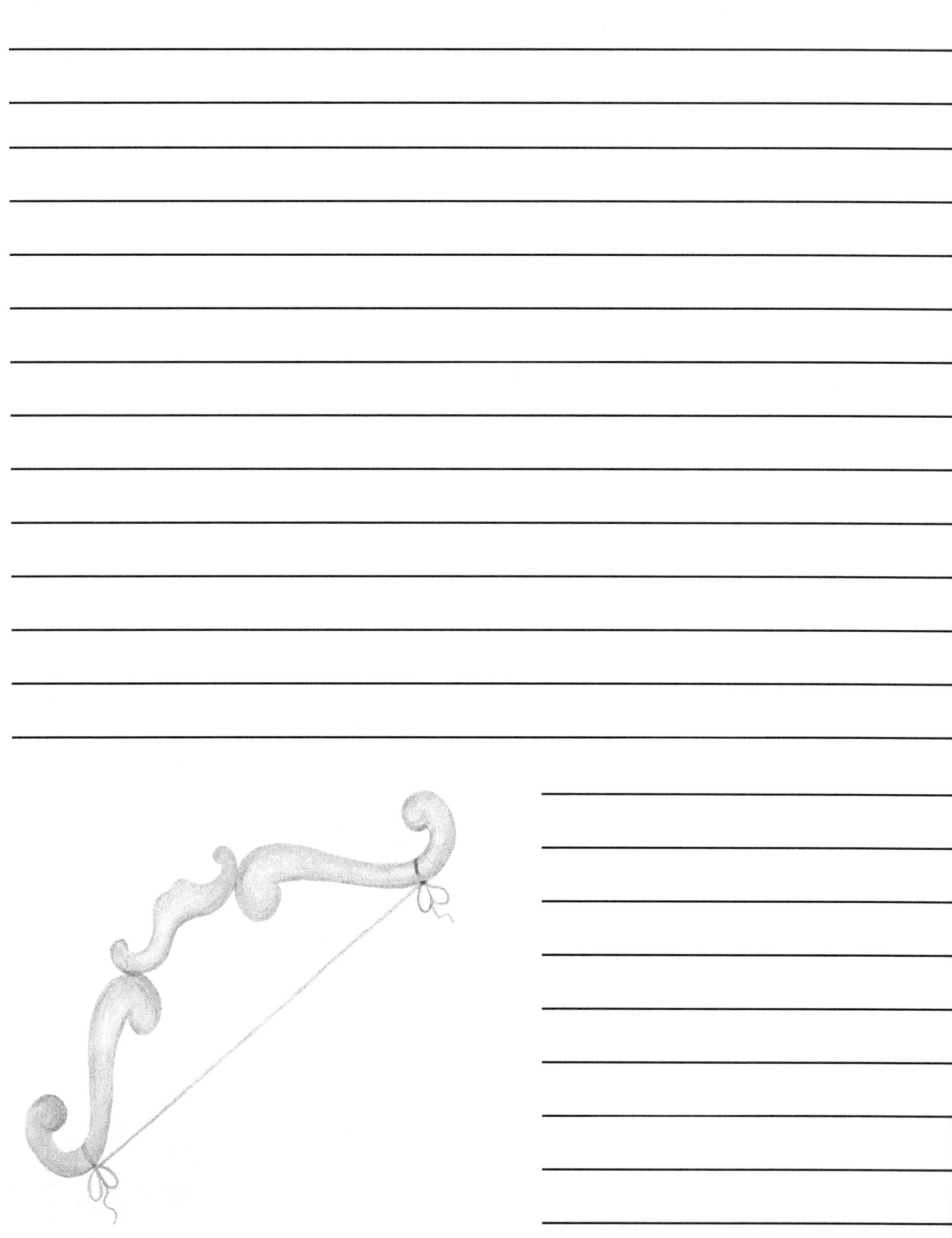

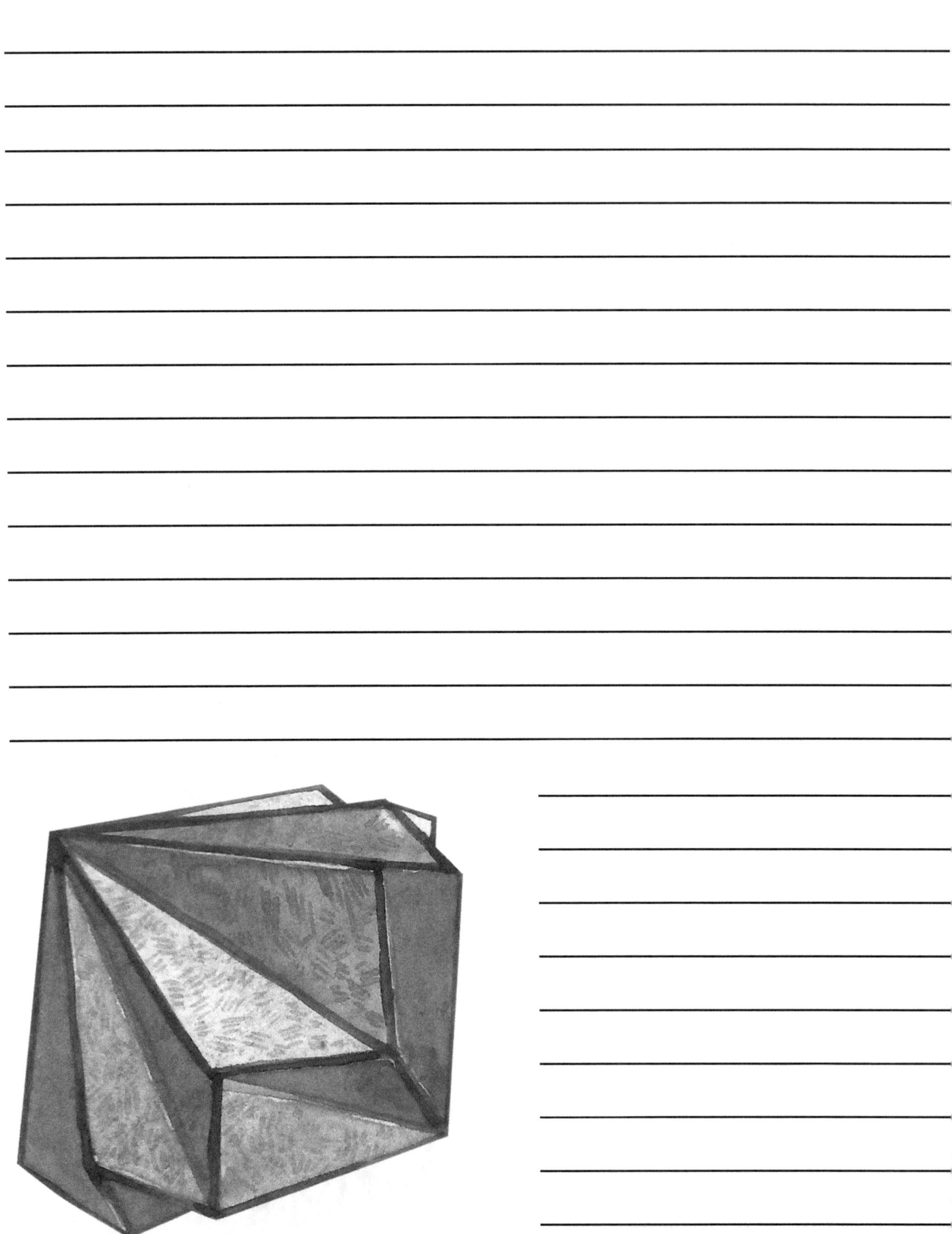

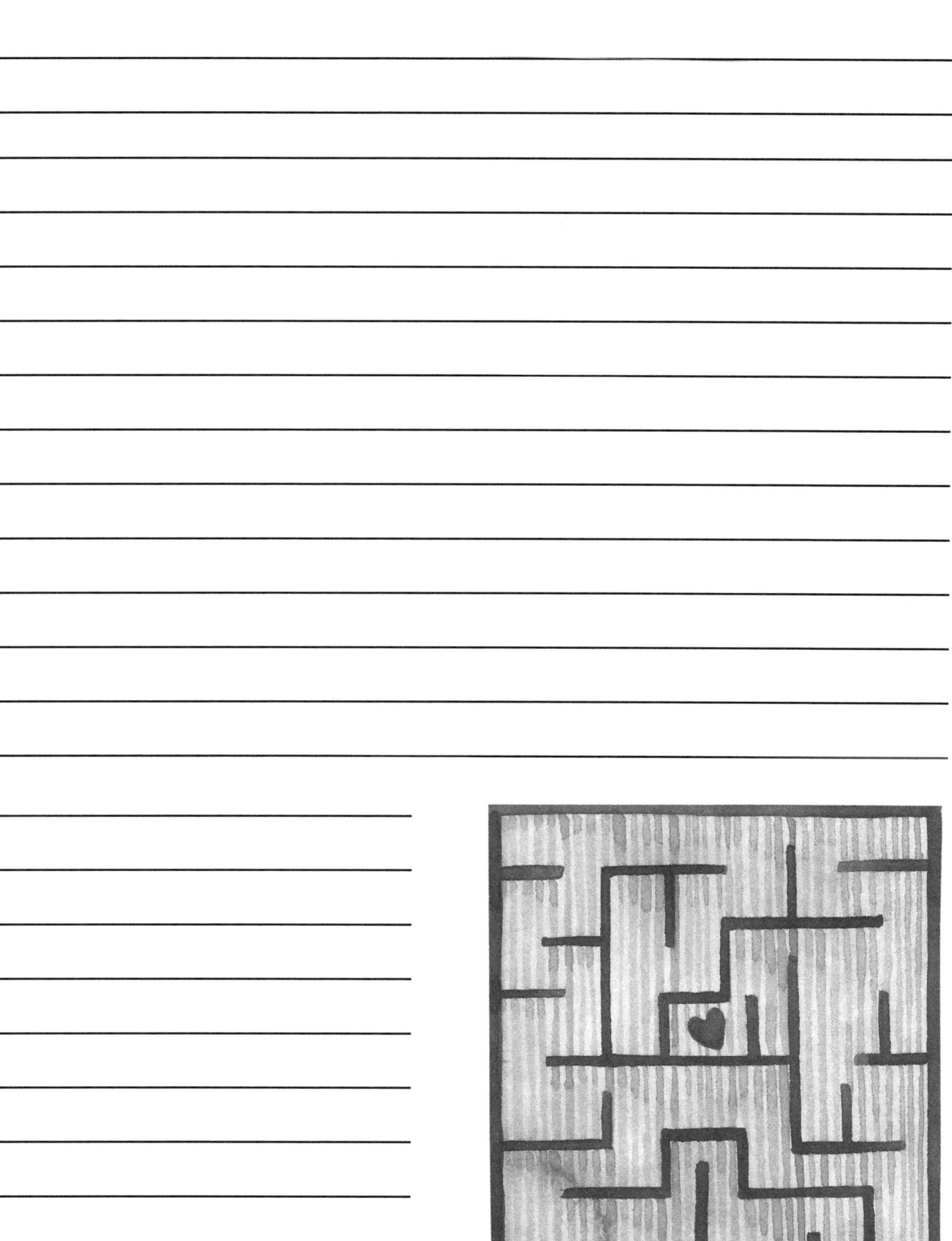

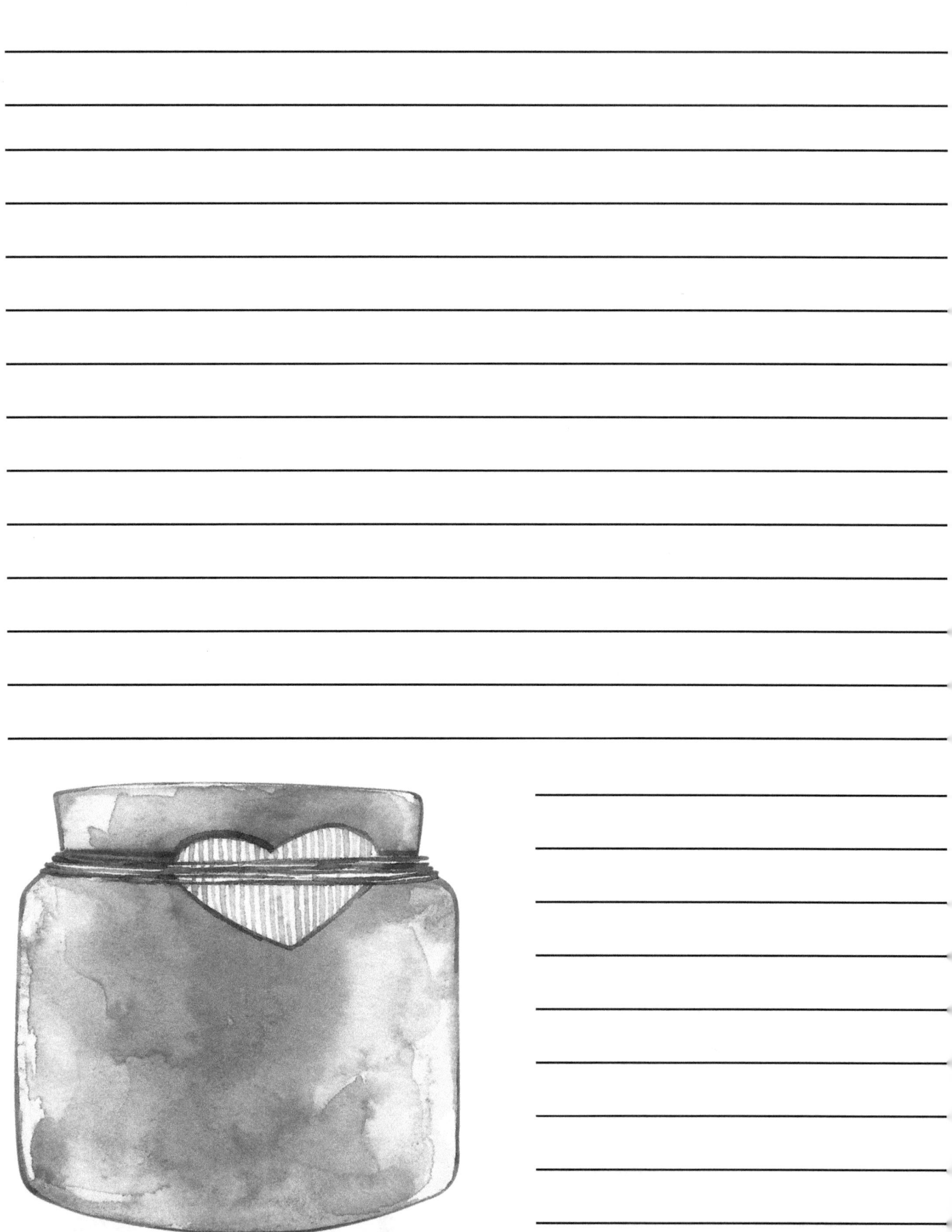

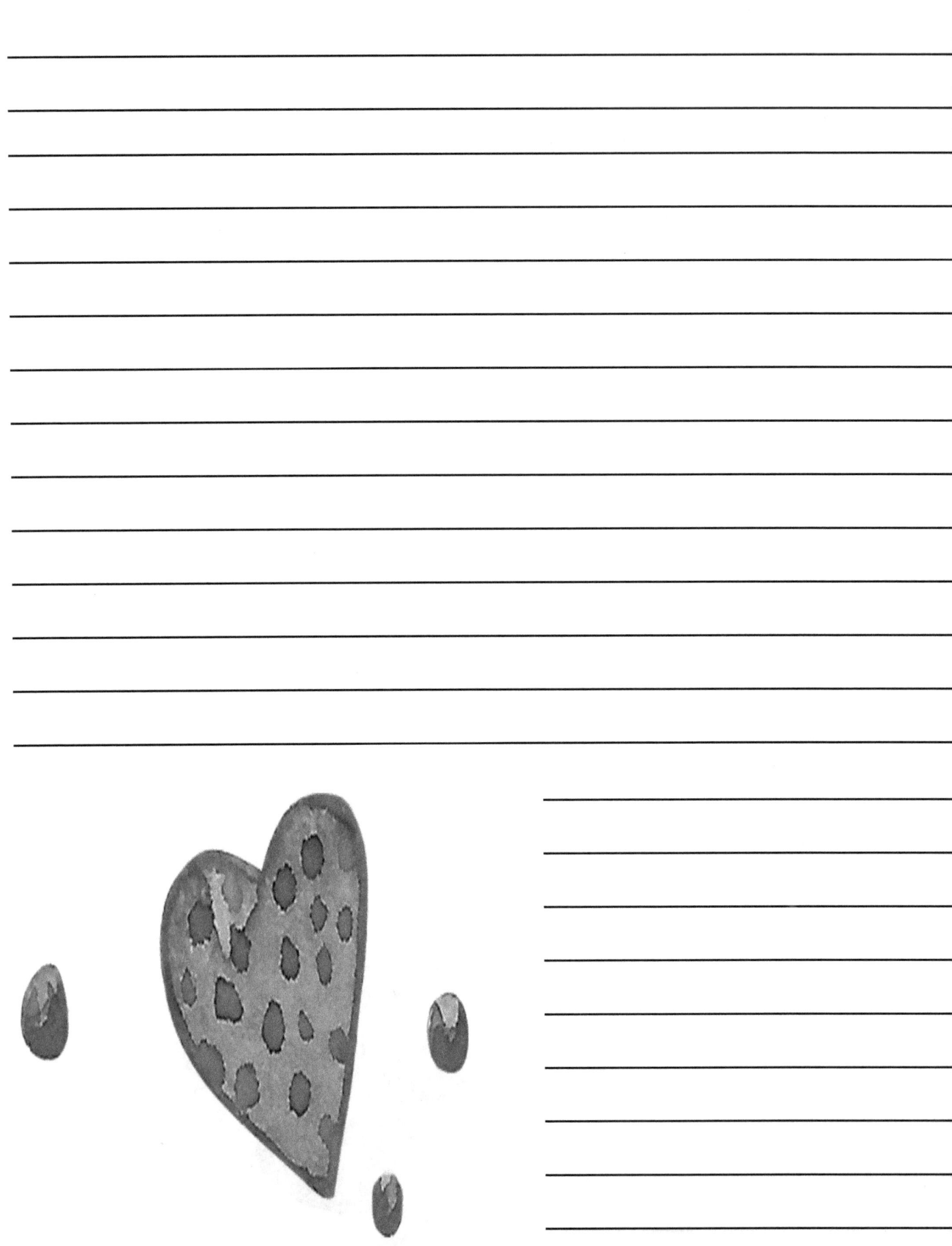

- Acts of Kindness Tracker -

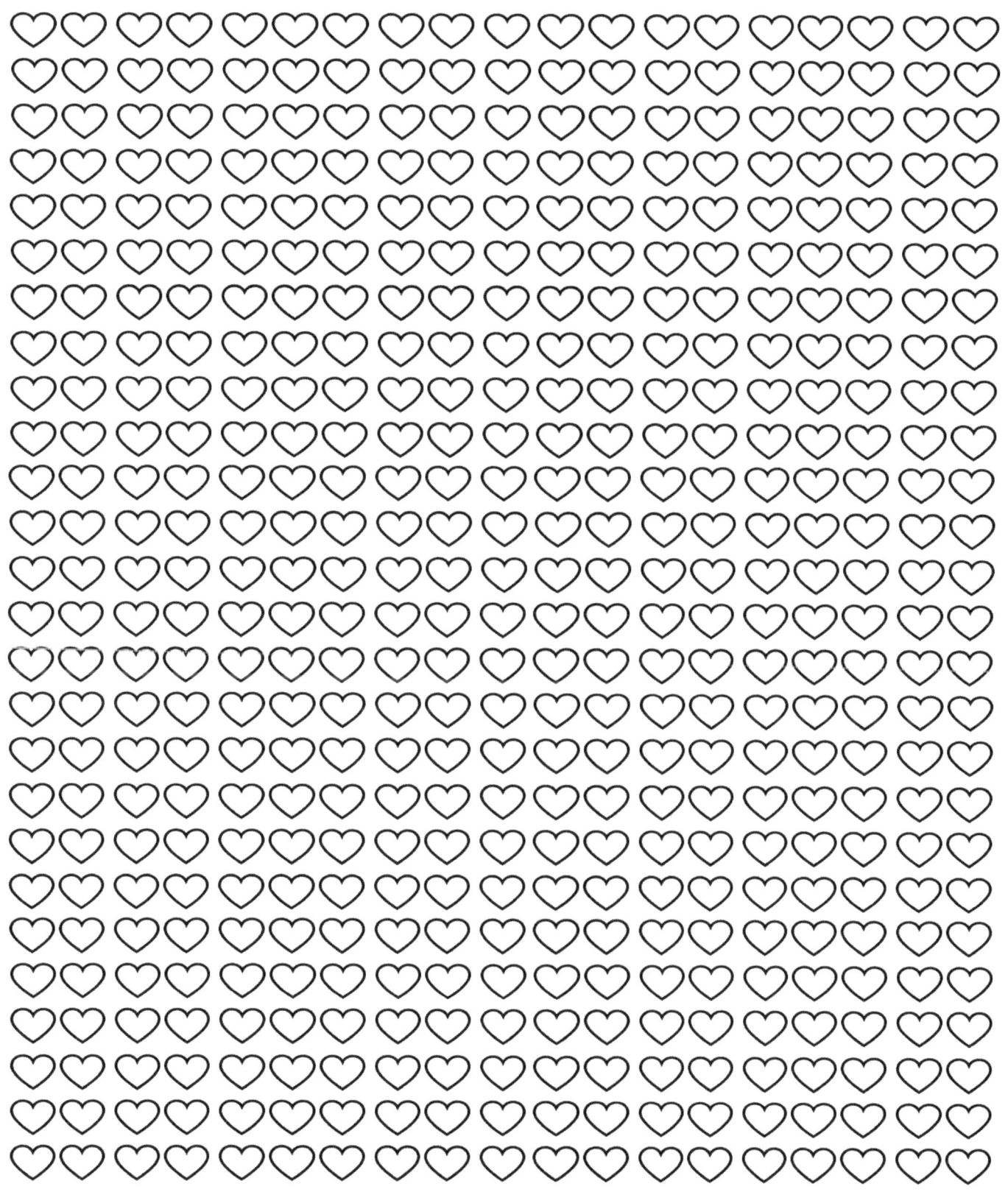

- Acts of Kindness Tracker -

- Acts of Kindness Tracker -

Notes

Notes

Notes

CPSIA information can be obtained
at www.ICGtesting.com
Printed in the USA
BVHW051936220221
600779BV00002B/65